FOUNDATIONS OF THE PSYCHOLOGICAL INTERVENTION

Foundations of the Psychological Intervention presents a new General Theory for Psychological Intervention (GTPI), delving into how its methodology can be applied across diverse psychological contexts.

Rooted in semiotic cultural psychology and guided by the GTPI framework, this book offers a cohesive perspective of psychology, addressing the prevailing fragmentation evident in various domains of psychology, such as health, sports, forensic, organizational, and clinical psychology. The framework establishes a foundation of methods and techniques that render psychological interventions applicable across various domains, substantiated by concrete examples from different areas. With chapters revolving around theories of action, change, and client dynamics, this groundbreaking work provides both a conceptual and methodological structure to underpin domain-specific theories and methodologies, thereby strengthening the conceptual links among distinct domains of psychology.

As one of the first works to develop a theory and method of intervention across multiple psychological domains, this book will be of interest to postgraduate students and researchers specializing in cultural psychology, clinical psychology, health psychology, and the philosophy of psychology. Moreover, it serves as a useful reading for practicing psychologists and psychology professionals.

Sergio Salvatore is Professor of Dynamic Psychology at the Department of Human and Social Sciences, Università del Salento, Italy.

Barbara Cordella is Psychotherapist and Assistant Professor of Clinical Psychology at the Department of Dynamic and Clinical Psychology and Health Studies, Sapienza University of Rome, Italy.

FOUNDATIONS OF THE PSYCHOLOGICAL INTERVENTION

A Unifying Theoretical and Methodological Framework

Sergio Salvatore
Barbara Cordella

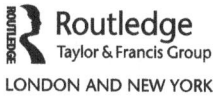

Routledge
Taylor & Francis Group

LONDON AND NEW YORK

Designed cover image: tbc

First published 2024
by Routledge
4 Park Square, Milton Park, Abingdon, Oxon OX14 4RN

and by Routledge
605 Third Avenue, New York, NY 10158

Routledge is an imprint of the Taylor & Francis Group, an informa business

British Library Cataloguing-in-Publication Data
A catalogue record for this book is available from the British Library

ISBN: 978-1-032-58271-9 (hbk)
ISBN: 978-1-032-58270-2 (pbk)
ISBN: 978-1-003-44936-2 (ebk)

DOI: 10.4324/9781003449362

Typeset in Galliard
by Apex CoVantage, LLC

CONTENTS

FIGURES

TABLES

FOREWORD

From A to A to A: abstraction as the key to application, which is aesthetic

This book carries with it a simple – yet profound – message for all the people who want to develop successful intervention programs. The message is – *in order to apply something in practice and succeed, the intervener needs to think.* To think means to consider the intervention plan systemically, abstractly, and strategically. As it happens in irreversible time – an intervention when it is made to happen cannot be taken back – it relies fully on abduction as its inferential basis. And here is the difficulty – facing a new goal of intervention into a system not yet fully known, the intervener extrapolates by abductive reconstruction of success (or failure) of past similar cases. Yet similarity is not sameness – and the new intervention effort is a risky step. A theory of intervention is needed.

It is needed – but building a theory is not supported nor understood. In our present-day pragmatic contexts of over-politicized societies, thinking is no simple task. Thinking needs liberation from practical action demands in order to be practical in action. This seems to be either a paradox or a tautology – to be practical, one needs to be non-practical. Yet it is needed – for distancing from the current stated need for intervention here and now to the generalized thinking of how established systems operating in a steady state might handle an intervention effort. The likely first response is resistance and neutralization. The systems are conservative – not easy to change. But the interventionist is an action wo(man), not a philosopher! They want concrete results.

Yet it is precisely a general theory that is needed – and, therefore, the coverage in the present book is intellectually refreshing and – pragmatically discouraging. It demonstrates how intervention efforts must be made free of prevailing opinions and concentrate on a generalized understanding of the nature of the effort. The simple "we intervene → all gets better" is replaced by "one tries to intervene → triggers systemic resistances → if lucky, has success that might differ from the expected." Interventions give us surprises.

The General Theory of Psychological Intervention (GTPI) that is presented in this book to an international readership is the result of the authors' decades-long attempt to conceptualize psychological intervention from a psychological standpoint. They considered psychological professional action not only as a way of *using* psychological scientific knowledge but also as an *object* of that knowledge. This creates a constructive duality – in order to use any object, the object has to be abstracted out from its instrumental frame into an abstract concept so as to be brought forward to practice. When I am invited to vote in a democratically organized election (my act of voting is an object that is being used in power-making by the ones I vote for), I need to be convinced that the basic abstract principles of such democratic election are in place in the social system that invites or demands my participation. If not – I would not vote, or my vote would not represent anything. The disputes – usually after elections – about whether the election was fair (or "rigged") is an act of using the abstract moral evaluator that would either support (fair) or undermine ("rigged") the meaning system of the given society. The notion of *fairness* of elections is an abstract principle that is a result of the framing of the meaning of the elections, while the individual voter's act in these elections is a concrete symbolic step – should I put the voting bulletin into a box in the voting station, or into a garbage container outside of that station. The physical act is the same, the personal symbolic meaning vastly different, and the possible societal evaluation is potentially damning. The person can be mobbed by the volunteers who consider the use of the garbage bowl as a political dissident act – even if it was merely a case of absent-mindedness.

Human beings relate to one another – and with "society" – always in varied states of abstractive generalization. Human conduct is constantly changing – re-negotiated by the participants in their social roles. How that happens is very nicely summarized in Table 3.1 – where the trajectories move from the most mundane everyday events that can be – but need not be – linked with the intermediate and highest levels of meaning construction. Thus, considering the everyday non-abstract forms of meaning (Row 1), we can find a simple story of neighbors greeting one another at the garage door on a regular basis, leading to the ordinary judgment "my neighbor is a courteous person." In contrast, at Row 5 (level of hyper-generalized signs), the abstract description "acting according to justice is the right way" elaborated by the trust in agreement and confidence in surroundings that leads to human rights advocacy activities. If the rows in Table 3.1 were each homogeneous and co-present in the minds of people in a society, we would be dealing with a caste society where the Brahmins operate at the generalized philosophical level (Row 5) while ordinary people live according to the mundane daily meaning systems (Row 1).

Such a simple solution is not what we encounter in present-day societies. More realistic is looking at the moves in human discourses across the diagonal of Table 3.1 – interpreting the polite neighbor at the garage door as a potential co-believer in the human rights advocacy – and trying to recruit her (or him) to that worthy activity domain. And be surprised if this effort fails. It is here where the abstraction processes take place and where the success or failure of an intervention program is determined. An educator bringing to a village school a new progressive teaching method and explaining it to teachers who are affectively oriented to pupils' progress and agree that "new methods" are always a good idea might fail to follow through in the program through simple distrust (generalized sign) in the school as an institution. As a result, there will be many nice general talks between the teachers and the intervener – but no concrete actions as the particular semiotic trajectory is blocked.

This hypothetical walk-through of Table 3.1 leads to the general issue – what are the mechanisms for blocking or enabling the meaning abstraction processes that mediate the intervention efforts? This should be the frame for the flow of semiotic capital elaborated for intervention contexts in Chapter 6.

GTPI zooms into the locus where intervention needs to take place – at the intermediate flow of meaning construction that persons are involved in communal settings. A new notion – *semiotic capital* – is central to the authors' argument about the psychological intervention process. This notion is an analogy to its economic forebears – the notion of capital made world-famous by Karl Marx and related to political discourses over the last century. Yet it has a daily analog for our thinking today – news reports from the "capital market" where the flows of financial powers are being re-negotiated. But what kind of "flow" can we posit for the fate of the *semiotic* capital? Can signs of various generality and form be traded, borrowed, loaned out (with interest) to the needy, and be "written off" when the actor on the semiotic capital market has to declare bankruptcy? In Chapter 6, the reader finds traces of this being possible – as the diagnosis of loss of semiotic capital in a given society is claimed. The large political gamble of co-existence within the European Union can lead to the semiotic impoverishment of the societies involved. But on what grounds can such claims be made?

The answer in terms of GTPI is in the development and dissemination of meanings – particularly the level of affective meanings – that constitute the basis for semiotic capital. What is at stake is the making of symbolic resources within social practices. Here, the processes of self-regulation – by persons, communities, and states – are the underlying mechanisms for the social maintenance of order and its possible change. Semiotic capital is produced, maintained, and

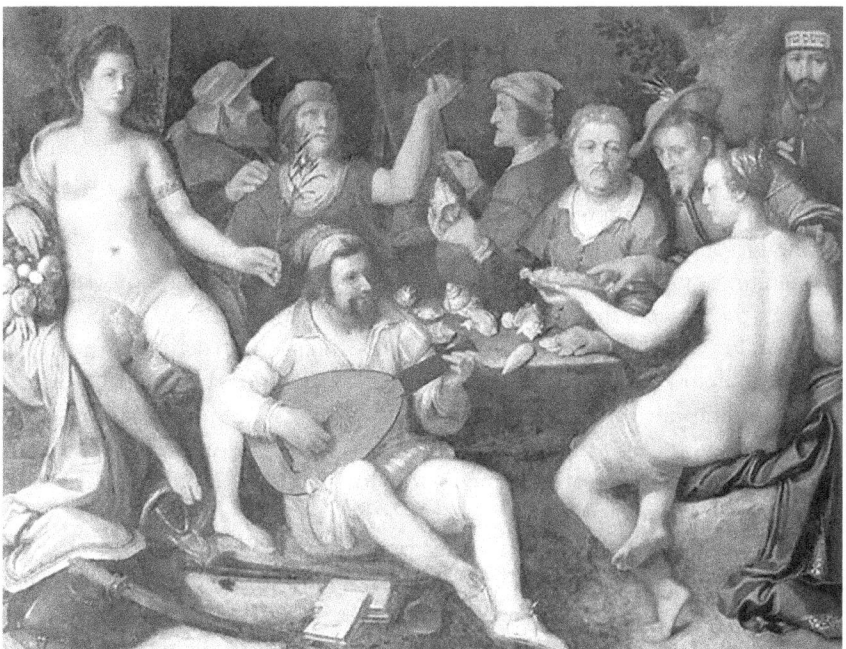

FIGURE 0.1 Allegory of Arts and Sciences

Source: Cornelis van Haarlem (1607)

lost within and through active social practice contexts within the community. These practices operate as incubators of new meanings – but how?

Possibly, an answer to this question is in the widespread use of allegories. These are hyper-generalized abstract meaning complexes that are encoded in ordinary cultural objects – paintings, songs, literary texts, fairy tales, popular street festivities, and, in sum, all kinds of social events that capture the imagination of the populace. Allegories are purposefully imprecise – vague and approximate – fields of signs that saturate society at the given time and guide the production of new meanings (Valsiner, 2023). They are hyper-generalized guidance devices for ordinary living – hence produced for the incubation of symbolic resources.

Figure 0.1 is an allegorical painting from the year 1607 by Dutch painter Cornelis van Haarlem. While labeled – *Allegory of Arts and Sciences* – it is a group portrait of the shell collector Jan Govertsz van der Aar, art writer Karel van Mander, engravings maker Hendrick Goltzius, and Jan Pieterszoon Sweelinck – all prominent personages in the beginning of the 17th century Low Countries. Hence, the manifest content of Figure 0.1 is that of a mundane portrait – a source of a depiction of the persons listed not available to us over centuries. Yet the whole context of the painting rises above the ordinary – the naked muses of art join the merrymaking of all with the focus on the natural science (shell collection) in the center. The whole of the painting guides the viewer towards hyper-generalized (therefore non-verbal) meaning-making of science as art that is accomplished through acceptance of ordinary human gatherings with music. The mundane and the abstract lead to the generalization of the meaning beyond the immediate information given.

The history of European art is filled with paintings similar to Figure 0.1 – all operating on the principle of going – in suggested meanings construction – between the objects that are depicted on the canvas. Likewise, in poetry, one finds – in between the lines – guidance for meaning construction of the hyper-generalized kind. Dante Alighieri's *Commedia* has, since the year 1324, invigorated generations of Italians in their search for their personal meanings using the emerging Italian language and establishing it as a beautiful vehicle for national identity. These are the incubators for symbolic resources – as equivalent to the semiotic capital.

Allegoric devices operate across historical time – they are functional over centuries. Their power is in their aboutness – they kind of "give" their user a meaning, yet they do not "give" but guide the user to saturate their external frame with personal meanings. Listening to the music of Beethoven – created at the beginning of the 19th century – relates to us in the 21st century by triggering our affective meaning construction processes. Our personal lives of 21st-century technologies become combined with 19th-century affective musical feelings. The personal bricolage of identity is thus guided by centuries past together with anticipations for the next year to come.

So – if we take GTPI seriously – which I strongly recommend to the readers of this book – a number of somewhat surprising necessities emerge for anybody who wants to make societal change. Abstract thinking is the prerequisite for any application of know-how – always in a new context. Furthermore – abstract thinking needs to consider the cultural history of the incubators of symbolic resources – and here, the role of aesthetic objects as a tool for interventions becomes valuable. The readers can understand that through the whole of this book.

Jaan Valsiner September 2023
Chapel Hill, NC

Reference

Valsiner, J. (2023). Creating glory out of miseries: Anatomy of the making of visual allegories. In J. Valsiner (Ed.), *Sensuous unity of art and science: The times of Rudolf II* (pp. 95–114). Information Age Publishers.

INTRODUCTION

The scientific-professional system of psychology has been working hard to empower its capacity to help address the many challenges that contemporary society is called on to tackle. The idea that prompted us to write this book is that the efforts that psychology is making in that direction have to be supported by reflective thinking and theoretical development of the fundamentals of intervention.

To develop its utility and appropriateness to demands and needs that individuals and social groups address to it, psychology needs to clarify to itself what the psychological function is and, therefore, what it can offer society. It is by anchoring itself in a solid, shared conception of the relationship between scientific knowledge and professional action that psychology can empower its capacity for innovation and for building credible and efficacious responses to the new forms of social demand.

With this book, we aim to make a contribution in that direction. In the following pages, the reader will find the outlines of a general model of psychological professional function – what we have called the General Theory of Psychological Intervention (GTPI). The GTPI is the result of our attempt to conceptualize psychological intervention from a psychological perspective: we considered professional psychological action not only as a way of using psychological scientific knowledge but also as an object of that knowledge. The GTPI is thus a *psychological theory* of psychological intervention.

We are fully aware that any attempt to arrive at a unified theory of the variegated archipelago of professional psychological practices is doomed to failure even before it is born when understood in reductionist and homogenizing terms. The plurality and heterogeneity of the levels and spheres of psychologists' actions, of the phenomena in relation to which they are called

DOI: 10.4324/9781003449362-1

upon to operate, does not allow one to think of the general theory of intervention in terms of identifying common elements that cut across the various forms of professional practice. Our idea of general theory is different. It is based on abstraction: the definition of a conceptual model of superordinate logical level – a meta-theory – that operates as a conceptual and methodological framework for sectoral theories, each focused on a field of intervention and/or type of phenomenon (e.g., psychotherapy, organizational counseling, community development). Thus, GTPI does not aim to replace sectorial theories by reducing them to what they have in common – on the contrary, the intent is to enhance the theories related to different contexts of professional action through their inscription in a general theoretical framework that facilitates the recognition of the conceptual links that exist between them and with the fundamental concepts of psychology as the science of mind and subjectivity.

We are certainly not the first to affirm the need for an organic perspective of the professional function. Think, just to give some examples, of the historical-epistemological reading proposed by Gaj (2009), the construction of a grid through which to put different therapeutic approaches in dialogue (Cionini, 2001), or the proposal to integrate different perspectives to address specific problems (Ivaldi, 2016).

Our attempt is part of a tradition of thought developing in Italian academic psychology since the mid-1980s on the impulse of Renzo Carli, who proposed to give theoretical and methodological grounding to psychological intervention (Carli, 1988; Carli & Paniccia, 1999, 2003; Circolo del Cedro, 1992; Grasso & Stampa, 2014).

Rooted in that tradition of thought, this book represents the culmination of a path of thought that has engaged the two authors for a quarter of a century. Twenty-five years have passed since the publication of the first volume in which Massimo Grasso, with one of us, addressed the issue of the psychological function and its object (Grasso & Salvatore, 1997). A few years later, the volumes *L'intervento in psicologia clinica* (Grasso et al., 2003) and *Metodologia dell'intervento in psicologia clinica* (Cordella et al., 2004) proposed a systematic examination of the theoretical, methodological, and technique-theory dimensions of psychological intervention, with particular reference to the clinical setting; an examination further developed in subsequent editions of the texts (Grasso et al., 2016; Cordella et al., 2022). In parallel, *L'intervento psicologico per la scuola. Modelli, metodi e strumenti* (Salvatore & Scotto di Carlo, 2005) constituted a first step in the direction of the elaboration of a unified model of the intervention – of its object, of the relationship with its user, of the dynamics and forms of change, and of ways to nurture it. The next step was taken with *L'intervento psicologico* (Salvatore, 2016a), which generalized the intervention model, initially elaborated with reference to the school context, to the whole of professional action.

With this volume, we take another step in this journey. It represents the English version of a book published in 2022 in Italian [*L'intervento psicologico*, Il Mulino]. The current text presents only marginal changes with respect to the Italian version, introduced to make it consistent with the international readership. In the pages that follow, the reader will find a comprehensive reformulation and systematization of the main themes of psychological intervention due to an innovative conception of the mind, subjectivity, and human relationships based on the integration of psychoanalytic theory, *embodied cognition*, and semiotic cultural psychology (Bruner, 1990; Salvatore & Freda, 2011; Salvatore, 2018; Valsiner, 2014). At the core of this conception is the idea that psychological processes – feeling, thinking, communicating, acting – are the ways through which the subject makes sense of experience. The focus of the psychological study of the human being is thus the dynamic of sensemaking. What characterizes this dynamic is its embodied nature and its affective foundation. Sensemaking is more than processing information – it is giving the content of experience to being-in-the-world in terms of the lived form of one's corporeality, as it is given in the moment-by-moment relationship to the world.

Adopting this conception as its foundation, GTPI assumes human interpretive activity as the (theoretical) *object* of psychological intervention and consistently draws from this assumption the foundational dimensions of psychological intervention: the *change* that the intervention proposes to promote, the *action* through which the psychologist pursues it, and the relationship with the *client*, which constitutes the context within which the action is performed and its results find value.

The book is organized into six chapters. The first acts as an overture. It introduces GTPI, discussing some of the epistemological and theoretical premises on which it is based – the conception of scientific knowledge, the relationship between scientific knowledge and intervention, and how to understand the unity to which GTPI aspires. In Chapter 2, the proposal of the dynamics of sensemaking as a metatheoretical object of psychological intervention is explored. This is done by presenting a general model of the dynamics of sensemaking, which is offered as a conceptual reference for the discussions in subsequent chapters. Parts of this chapter take up and develop parts of Chapter 3 of a recently published volume by one of the authors and colleagues, focusing on cultural psychological theory and its implications in the socio-political field (Cremaschi et al., 2021). Chapter 3 focuses on the change that psychological intervention aims to promote. The proposed model of change is an attempt to open the black box – that is, to understand not only the content of the change and the conditions that induce it but also the underpinning mechanism. Chapter 4 is devoted to a discussion of the operations and devices that the psychologist can deploy to determine the conditions that induce change. In this context, specific attention is given to conceptualizing the relationship between the general value of the scientific knowledge that the psychologist uses within and as a function of the context of intervention and the contingent nature of the latter. Chapter 5 delves into the various issues related to the relationship with the client. The concepts of request and demand and the forms of their development are discussed. The issue of the value of the intervention and the different forms of responsibility that the psychologist assumes with respect to it are also addressed. Chapter 6 presents elaborations of GTPI within domains of intervention covering the different levels of professional action, from the individual to the macro-social level. The intent of that concluding chapter is to show how the abstract nature of GTPI does not hinder, but on the contrary, fosters, the development of interpretive models and intervention strategies capable of providing feasible and appropriate responses to the plurality of issues on which psychology can provide its contribution. For sure, we are not the first to assert that there is nothing more practical than a good theory.

We would like to conclude these introductory pages by expressing our thanks.

We are grateful to our students. This book carries with it endless traces of the discussions we had with them, the changes and reworking we were forced to do in response to their comments, requests for clarification, objections, and reformulations.

We are grateful to Matteo Reho for his precious support in the translation from the Italian version.

We are grateful to Raffaele De Luca Picione, Santo Di Nuovo, Arianna Palmieri, and Giampaolo Salvatore for their encouragement, comments, suggestions, and criticisms. This book would have been different, for the worse, had it not been able to take advantage of their generous support.

We are grateful to Daniele Malaguti, our editor (of the Italian version), for his unfailing support and for the courtesy with which he offered it to us. On several occasions, we had the comforting feeling that the book was a fixed point in his mind even when it worked like a flickering light bulb in ours.

We are grateful to Jaan Valsiner, whose Preface enriches the volume and witnesses the fecundity and beauty of a scientific dialogue that has been alive for two decades.

Our thoughts, at once of gratitude, affection, and sadness go to Renzo Carli. He left us just as we were arranging to write the first Italian version of the volume. We do not know how much he would have agreed with what we have come to propose; we are sure, however, that he would have grasped how every single page of this book finds its source of inspiration in his teaching.

1

THE GENERAL THEORY OF PSYCHOLOGICAL INTERVENTION

The General Theory of Psychological Intervention (GTPI) refers to the conceptualization of the psychologist's intervention as a function of the field conditions (interpersonal, sociocultural, institutional) within which it unfolds as a competent action seeking to generate value for the user.

Generally speaking, psychological intervention can be understood as a form of human activity characterized by the fact that someone (the psychologist) exercises his or her scientifically grounded knowledge to perform an action aimed at obtaining a result that generates value for someone else (the client). From this general definition, we deduce the issues around which GTPI is structured. These issues, taken together, map the components of professional action.

The first and foundational question that GTPI addresses is the domain of the intervention competence: what defines the intervention as *psychological*? How does it differ from practices of other kinds? Since psychological intervention is grounded in psychological scientific knowledge, the answer to these questions requires a conceptualization of the object of the psychological science. In what follows, we will refer to this area as the *theory of the object*: the modeling of the class of phenomena to which scientific psychological knowledge refers.

The second issue concerns the process by which the intervention produces the desired outcome. The *theory of the change* is the part of GTPI that aims at understanding this process from a psychological perspective. What changes occur in the psychological intervention? Under what conditions and through what mechanisms does this happen?

The third question concerns the psychologist's action – the way he or she activates and regulates the process of change: what vectors does the psychologist

DOI: 10.4324/9781003449362-2

use to trigger, feed, and channel the mechanisms underlying change? What devices mediate the mobilization of these vectors? This is the area of GTPI that we will refer to with the term the *theory of the action*.

The fourth issue recalled by the general definition concerns the fact that intervention involves a user. The *theory of the client* is the area of GTPI that conceptualizes the sociocultural and psychosocial process underlying the social and subjective construction of the client. It aims at answering questions such as: what is the psychological process underlying the client's request to the psychologist? What is the relationship between that process and the intervention? What relationship exists between the client's goals, the objectives of the intervention, and the value the latter generates for the client?

Theory of the object, theory of the change, theory of the action, and theory of the client are the four components of GTPI. Each of these theories will be the subject of one of the following chapters. Preliminarily, we devote this chapter to the discussion of two epistemological assumptions that inform the entire conceptual-methodological edifice that this book proposes – the idea of the unity of psychological science and the dialectical link between scientific knowledge and professional practice.

1 One hundred thousand, no one or one?[1]

Professional action selects events and situations on which to operate based on the understanding that scientific knowledge about them offers. To give just a few examples, one finds it obvious that the psychologist deals with personality disorders, learning problems, personnel selection, school dropouts, and community interventions since it is assumed that psychology offers the basis of scientific understanding to intervene in such phenomena.

Therefore, it is important to understand what the sphere of competence of psychology is and how it is defined – namely, the conceptual premises based on which certain phenomena are considered the object of psychological science and, thus, of the professional action related to that system of knowledge.

One hundred thousand

Contemporary psychology is concerned with a plethora of phenomena spanning virtually every sphere of human activity. The constructs through which these phenomena are interpreted are equally heterogeneous – for example, personality, attachment, cognitive styles, motivation, metacognition, heuristics, attitudes, leadership, sense of community, trust, and so on. A common denominator underlying this heterogeneity can nevertheless be traced: psychological constructs generally refer to particular forms of mental activity – to the characteristics/modes of its functioning, its products, and behavioral or neurobiological correlates. However, the conceptual link between different constructs, especially those relating to different levels – individual, group, social – and domains – e.g., psychotherapy, health, schooling, sports, marketing – is generally weak, when not entirely absent. As a result of this, contemporary psychology, rather than a unified doctrinal corpus, appears to be a web of pieces of disciplinary knowledge to be viewed in the plural – psychological sciences rather than psychological science.

At the first level of analysis, we can observe that the pluralism and separateness of psychological knowledge is the precipitate of the progressive reduction in the scope of theories that has marked the evolution of the discipline since the 1960s (e.g., Valsiner, 2007). Contemporary psychology today is populated by models of limited range – namely, constructs developed to conceptualize circumscribed phenomenal domains or even specific phenomena. Attachment styles, core values, and support for democracy are examples of mid-range constructs used within a circumscribed phenomenal domain: individual and interpersonal mental functioning, social behavior, and political behavior, respectively. Other constructs – e.g., therapeutic alliance, burn out, sense of community – are related to even more specific phenomenal domains: psychotherapy, certain forms of work activity, and community bonds.

The existence of medium and short-range theories is not in itself a negative fact; on the contrary, it is indicative of the articulation and development of a scientific discipline and its ability to broaden and deepen its areas of interest. Generally, however, it is the fundamental theory that grounds, guides, and provides the method, frameworks, and basic categories needed by subdisciplines if they are to develop. The same cannot be said for psychology. Medium- and short-range psychological constructs maintain a weak, or even very weak, connection with the fundamental concepts of the discipline. This is reflected in the constructs' tendency to become autonomous and to be used as if they were primitive concepts endowed with meaning in themselves rather than in relation to the more general theoretical framework. The consequence of this is that the landscape of contemporary psychology resembles Italy before the Risorgimento: an assemblage of duchies, principalities, and kingdoms, each operating as an autonomous entity.

To delve into the reasons behind this state of contemporary psychology would be beyond the scope of this book and, even more, beyond the writers' expertise. We, therefore, confine ourselves to recalling some factors that have played a role in determining the current geography of the discipline. On the one hand, the role played by the powerful advancement of methods and tools of analysis must be acknowledged. The technical and technological apparatus of research has grown significantly, becoming more specialized and reflecting the peculiarities of the different domains of investigation. As a result, the fields of analysis have multiplied and drifted apart, eventually becoming separate territories with almost no transversal links. Today, the vast majority of researchers (and professionals) specialize in one or two areas, acquiring advanced knowledge and skills in the languages, methods, tools, and theories that substantiate that domain. The knowledge and skills developed in other domains are often so vastly different as to be practically irrelevant, or at least that is how they are thought to be. For example, those who carry out research in psychotherapy do so with theories, methods, and tools that have only marginal overlap with the theories, methods, and tools used by those who deal, for example, with the cognitive processes underlying decision-making or voting behavior, community interventions, and so on. Moreover, this separation is sanctioned and further nurtured by a clear separation between scientific communities, each endowed with its own organizational structures, venues, and communication tools (conferences, journals, scientific associations).

It should be noted, however, that technical progress has also characterized other sciences – in some cases probably even more markedly – without, however, producing any compartmentalization effects. In psychology, such effects have occurred because the centrifugal drive induced by technical development has been further fueled, rather than counterbalanced, by the empiricist view of scientific knowledge that has gradually taken over the discipline since the post-World War II period (Toomela & Valsiner, 2010). According to this view, scientific knowledge consists of the identification of empirical relationships among psychological constructs and between them and the phenomena being investigated, all through controlled procedures that can guarantee the reliability of results. A major implication of such a view is that it leads to the conception of psychological constructs in terms close to experience so that their meaning tends to be self-evident and thus objectifiable. Consider, for example, the concept of therapeutic alliance. This construct refers to certain characteristics (agreement on goals, quality of the bond, adherence to the role; cf. Bordin, 1979; Lingiardi, 2002) of the relationship between psychotherapist and patient. These characteristics, although in part not directly perceptible, are nevertheless definable in terms of concrete experiences, of self-evident meaning occurring within the exchange between therapist and patient. Similarly, the concept of a sense of community (Peterson et al., 2008) is defined as an internal state (a belief) that can be inferred from observable elements (the response to the scale used to measure the construct) and referable to an element (the community) that can equally be represented in factual terms – the set of people living in a given area.

The preference of empiricism for constructs close to experience has been accompanied by a downsizing of the role of abstract concepts – namely, concepts whose meaning is defined using theoretical frameworks rather than determined by factual content (Valsiner & Salvatore, 2012). Take the Gestalt notion of good form and closure (for a review, see Wagemans, 2018), Piagetian constructs of assimilation and accommodation (e.g., Piaget, 1936), notions of mediation (e.g., Vygotsky, 1934/1986), schema (Neisser, 1976), and liminality (Stenner, 2017): these constructs are abstract rather than empirical in nature; each can be used to conceptualize an infinity of phenomena, even very different at the empirical level. For example, the Piagetian concepts of assimilation and accommodation can be used to describe human thinking as well as organizational development. This is because abstract constructs are not defined in terms of empirical content but are grounded in the theoretical framework in which they are embedded. This does not mean that abstract constructs are anti-empirical; rather, it means that it is the theoretical framework of reference that, in grounding the definition of the abstract construct, also regulates the ways the empirical data are to be interpreted to produce information related to the construct. For example, continuing to refer to Piagetian constructs, it is not the child's behavior that defines the (empirical) meaning of assimilation, but the (theoretical) meaning of assimilation that allows the child's behavior to be interpreted in that sense (for a discussion of how abstract constructs can be empirically validated, see Salvatore & Valsiner, 2009, 2010).

It is not coincidental that the abstract concepts we have referred to were developed in a different historical period. Contemporary psychology has marginalized abstract concepts because they are not definable and measurable in terms of their empirical content but require the use of inferences, which, though disciplined by the theory, weaken the claim of research objectivity.

Now, there is a structural linkage between the centrality assumed by empirical constructs in psychology and the compartmentalization of the latter. The datum of experience belongs, by definition, to a context, and its immediate, self-evident meaning is the one it takes on in the context where it is needed. Attachment behavior occurs and is recognizable as such in the context of relationships with parents and significant persons, the therapeutic alliance in the context of psychotherapy, the sense of community in the context of relationship with one's community, and so on. The compartmentalization of psychology – psychotherapy, school psychology, hospital psychology, tourism psychology, etc. – thus finds its foundation and constraint in the centrality attributed to empirical concepts and the simultaneous marginalization of abstract constructs.

No one

Without disavowing the progress that contemporary psychology has made over the past half-century, our thesis is that its compartmentalization is a factor of structural weakness, decisively hindering the discipline's ability to produce theoretical innovation, professional empowerment, and social and institutional impact. This is for three fundamental reasons (for a discussion, see Salvatore, Ando', et al., 2022).

First, viewing psychology in the plural makes it subordinate to common sense. As we discussed previously, most psychological constructs find meaning because of the self-evidence of their factual content. This implies that psychological constructs are ultimately defined in terms of common sense, as it is the everyday language that determines their self-evident quality. Let us return to the examples given in the previous section: the meaning of constructs like attachment styles, therapeutic alliance, core values, support for democracy, burn out, and sense of community – and we might add emotion, motivation, aggression, dependency, and so on – comes from everyday language. Such constructs are not understood on the basis of theoretical premises proper to psychology but rather because of the practical knowledge that each member of the social group possesses as a result of his or her participation in the group's culture. On the other hand, if this were not the case, such constructs would not be self-evident, as is, in fact, the case with concepts such as proton, attractor, isomers, autopoiesis, endoplasmic reticulum, etc., the meaning of which is comprehensible only from within and by reason of the general theory of the scientific discipline they refer to (physics, chemistry, biology). The point is that the grounding of many psychological constructs in common sense comes at a high cost to the discipline and the profession: it makes scientific psychological knowledge – therefore professional action – ultimately take the form of an explication and systematization of the practical and implicit knowledge about subjectivity and human relationships active in the cultural environment that organizes the everyday thinking of people and institutions (Salvatore, 2016b – on the idea that much psychological knowledge is part of common sense, see Smedslund, 1988). This is true for any scientific field that moves within the realm of the human – but it is even more so for psychology, as the forms of naïve psychological knowledge (theory of mind, metacognition, narratives about the self) are the foundation of the mind and therefore of the ways humans exercise their subjectivity. Psychology should conceptualize, understand, and, in its professional component, interact dialectically with such ways rather than uncritically take them as its foundation.

Second, the compartmentalization of psychology results in a weakening of learning opportunities for psychologists. Sub-disciplinary fields tend to be closed communities of practice characterized by languages, technical apparatuses, traditions, standards, and rituals increasingly separate from each other. This limits and disincentivizes the possibility of cross-fertilization: opportunities to use information and knowledge produced in one field to enhance ways of working in other domains are severely limited. On the contrary, researchers and practitioners are incentivized to pursue their own advancement, thus the development of the system as a whole, in terms of a progressive increase in the specialization of their work. This runs along two mutually complementary paths: on the one hand, through the progressive differentiation of the phenomena of competence – see, for example, the tendency in the field of psychotherapy to identify specific treatments by a single disorder and even by subclasses of single disorders; on the other, an enhancement of the technical and technological content of the action – for example, increasingly sophisticated data analysis models and the use of apps and other devices derived from robotics and artificial intelligence. Of course, this is anything but a negative development. What is critical is the absence of a balance that would allow the drive for specialization to be integrated – and oriented – with the ability of specialisms to communicate with each other, in the perspective of the development of an overall framework that would further enhance their capacities for innovation and impact.

Third, compartmentalization both reflects and fosters psychology's subalternity to the social demand. The domains in which psychology is divided reflect how society is organized, separating the modes and processes of its reproduction into spheres of life and contexts of activity. Care, schooling, sports, tourism, and stages of the life cycle are not objects of nature endowed with their own ontological substance but social forms founded on and regulated by specific symbolic and institutional apparatuses subject to historical evolution. To the extent that psychology takes such social forms as its own target, it is, in fact, accepting that its scientific agenda, its project of development, depends on and is configured by the historical evolution of the ways society is segmented into spheres of activity and establishes a hierarchy of value among them. Needless to say, here, we do not intend to criticize the attention that psychology pays to the social question. Instead, we want to highlight the confusion between the useful and appreciable sensitivity to the problems that society poses to psychology and the tendency to design the present and future of psychological science – its disciplinary identity – in terms of the problems/constructions that society from time to time expresses, rather than in terms of the discipline's internal theoretical apparatus and lines of development. If you like, the confusion at stake is between a psychology *for* X (where X is the social phenomenon/sector – marketing, gambling, populism, addiction, pandemic) and a psychology *of* X, that is, a psychology that is understood, by psychologists primarily, as a discipline that has the social phenomenon/sector as its object.

One

Is there an alternative to the plural and compartmentalized definition of the object of psychology?

Our thesis is that such an alternative is possible and should be sought in the definition of a unified, abstract, and general object to be placed as the foundation and horizon of meaning of psychological science and professional action. This thesis underlies the structure of the entire book. We indicate its qualifying points in what follows, leaving the development of its implications to subsequent chapters.

As a premise, we would like to point out that the issue of the unification of psychology is not merely a philosophical matter, good for animating discussion among a small circle of specialists. The unification of psychology is a central crossroads in the development of scientific and professional psychology. Henriques (2011), one of the authors who has contributed most to the contemporary discussion on the topic, has pointed out that the unification of psychology serves to endow the discipline with the metatheoretical structure necessary to define the object of the discipline and to integrate key insights from the main perspectives so that cumulative knowledge might be possible.

First of all, it must be acknowledged that the way of understanding and pursuing the unification of psychology is anything but unified: efforts that have cyclically tried to address the fragmentation of psychology (e.g., Gaj, 2009; Henriques, 2011; Kimble, 1990; Mandler, 2011; Valsiner, 2009; Salvatore, 2017; Zagaria et al., 2020) follow different approaches, which are not always compatible with each other. In 2013, the Review of General Psychology devoted a special issue to the topic. The number (19) and variety of contributions hosted testify to the interest in the topic; at the same time, it is indicative of how complex the discussion is and how difficult it is to identify a unifying perspective. Most of the efforts start from the idea that the unification of psychology requires the adoption of the paradigmatic foundation of other sciences (for a different approach, based on the conceptual analysis of the ontological premises that ground current medium-range models, see Marsh & Boag, 2014). For example, Kimble (1990) identifies physics as the basis for the unification of psychology. In contrast, Lickliter and Honeycutt (2013), Melchert (2016), and more recently, Zagaria et al. (2020) propose the theory of evolution as the anchorage. However, such approaches have raised criticisms of reductionism (e.g., Green, 2015; Stam, 2004), ultimately claiming the need to elaborate the paradigmatic foundation from within the language of the discipline.

Our idea of unification lies within the latter endogenous logic. Obviously, the unified object cannot be defined at the empirical level – namely, by identifying what there is in common between the different phenomena tackled by psychology. Given the breadth of the discipline's areas of interest, this "bottom-up" search for the common denominator could only be doomed to failure: what do bullying and populist adherence, personality disorders, and customer satisfaction have in common empirically? The unitary object must therefore be identified through a different strategy in terms of generalizing abstraction (Salvatore & Valsiner, 2010). According to this strategy, the object of psychology should be understood as a general metatheoretical construct within which medium- and short-range constructs can be framed. In this way, empirical constructs do not lose relevance; on the contrary, they take on additional theoretical significance as they can be interpreted as local versions, in given contextual conditions and phenomenal domains, of the metatheoretical construct.

The general object is necessarily abstract, namely, devoid of empirical content. It is only on that condition, in fact, that it can operate as a metatheoretical framework for the potentially infinite class of phenomena and empirical constructs at the center of psychology's interest. Physics provides us with a paradigmatic example of generalizing abstraction. The apple falling on Newton's head, a skier leaving lines in the snow, the Earth with its orbit around the Sun, the vase shattering as it falls, and the flight of birds, while having no element of empirical resemblance, are all phenomena of interest to physics. This is because it interprets them in terms of generalizing abstraction: as local forms, contingent on certain contextual conditions, of the same fundamental dynamic, which is gravity.

2 The object of psychology as a metatheoretical construct

Phenomenon, process, and fundamental dynamic

The proposal outlined previously to define the object of psychology in terms of a generalizing abstraction is based on a theoretical assumption that is worth making explicit: the field conception of psychological processes. This conception is based on the distinction between *phenomenon, process,* and *fundamental dynamic.*

The *phenomenon* is what happens: a state of things that the observer experiences directly or indirectly, for example, an event, an utterance, or a behavior. The phenomenon occurs in a space and in a time within a given context of human activity (interpersonal relationships, school, work environment, sporting activity, public sphere) and takes on meaning because of the sociocultural norms that embody the common sense regulating that context. Mental suffering, gambling, school dropout, organizational conflict, anti-migrant narratives, and adherence to vaccination campaigns are examples of phenomena of interest to psychology, defined and interpreted by common sense. From the perspective of psychology, each phenomenon can be modeled as the manifestation of an underlying psychological process, active within the context of human activity where the phenomenon is manifested.

The *psychological process* is not immediately observable; by definition – it is latent. This is not because it is "hidden"; it is latent because it consists of a set of dynamic relationships (unfolding, reproducing and/or changing over time) among elements. In other words, the process is an organization capable of reproducing itself over time (for a discussion of organization as a unit of analysis in psychology, see Mandler, 2011). Consequently, to represent a process, one needs ad hoc constructs arranged to map not individual aspects but relationships and their variation over time (Salvatore & Tschacher, 2012).

Incidentally, what has just been said offers a further critical argument toward atheoretical empiricism as the foundation of psychology (without, however, implying a renunciation of empiricism): the dynamic relations that characterize a process can be mapped empirically – namely, they can be detected and measured; however, as the number of possible relations among relevant aspects is infinite, one can only select the potentially relevant relations if one has a theoretical model of the psychological process. And this means that in order to study a process scientifically, it is not enough to rely on empirical evidence. One also needs a theoretical model that allows one to *construct* the empirical data – that is, to identify the relevant relationships to be empirically detected.

In summary, the process is the explanatory premise (*explanans*) in terms of which the phenomenon (*explanandum*) is modeled psychologically. While the latter is defined in terms of common sense, the process is a scientifically grounded interpretation of the phenomenon. Here is where the notion of the field comes in: *psychological processes are to be conceptualized as local versions (instantiations) of a single fundamental dynamic* (henceforth, when the reference is clear, just "dynamic"), of which the modeling is the core purpose of psychological science – that is, its theoretical object. For example, the clinical exchange (phenomenon) is characterized by a cyclical pattern (process), which constitutes the way the dynamic of signification (fundamental dynamic) is instantiated in the field conditions characterizing the context of human interaction making up psychotherapy (see Chapter 6).

In general and abstract terms, given a class of elements, the dynamic can be defined as the bounded space of possible evolutive trajectories of the relationships among the elements of the class (Salvatore, 2018). The dynamic, then, is not a state of affairs but a potentiality (for a discussion of the ontology of potentiality, see Fronterotta et al., 2018); it is not something that happens – processes (i.e., the single evolutive trajectories) are what come into existence, as the specific and particular forms that dynamic takes due to field conditions. More specifically, each field imposes constraints on the fundamental dynamic and thereby a reduction of its potentialities, from which the local process emerges (Salvatore, De Luca Picione, et al., 2022). Thus, the dynamic is an abstract entity, theoretical in nature, void of empirical content. Thanks to it, however, psychological processes can be generalized and conceptualized in unified terms – that is, understood as forms that, although different in their empirical content, emerge from the same field of potentiality.

One final remark in closing this paragraph. Generalizing abstraction represents a different approach from the efforts to build general theories that aim at attributing psychological phenomena to supposed causal mechanisms detected by basic sciences (particularly biology, cf. Lickliter & Honeycutt, 2013; but also physics, cf. Kimble, 1990). By contrast, generalizing abstraction implies an anti-reductionist approach. This is because the fundamental dynamic is conceived not as a lower logical explanatory level but as the superordinate theoretical framework that provides the general semantics for interpreting phenomena from a specifically psychological perspective. We recognize that this way of conceiving psychology, characterized by the recovery of its abstract and theoretical depth, diverges from contemporary mainstream orientations. However, it is rooted in the rich tradition of 20th-century psychology, characterized by the development of general theories: Gestalt theory, Behaviorism, Cognitivism, and Cultural psychology. Piaget's work is, in this sense, paradigmatic. Piagetian theory, in fact, requires a twofold level of reading. On the first level, the theory of the ontogeny of thought is a medium-range theory (of how the child's cognitive system emerges and develops). However, through this domain theory, Piaget pursued a more general scientific goal: the modeling of the fundamental cognitive dynamic that characterizes living systems.

Why make things complicated?

The reader may find it surprising to encounter, in a book that sets out to conceptualize professional intervention, an undoubtedly complicated and abstract theoretical discussion about the unification of the object of the discipline. We believe, however, that there are three good reasons to consider this discussion relevant.

Firstly, the field model of the psychological object is a useful tool to resist the pressure of common sense that influences psychological research and the psychological profession ubiquitously. Conceiving the psychological object in abstract and meta-empirical terms enhances the separation and autonomy of psychological language from common sense. Physics is there to demonstrate that a theoretically strong discipline that proceeds by reason of its own language and developmental project does not thereby isolate itself from the world – on the contrary, the epistemological autonomy of physics is the condition of its extraordinary ability to produce technological spillovers in society.

Secondly, the definition of a single object favors the interpretation of emerging phenomena, thus the possibility of extending the areas of intervention as a result of the crises that people, groups, and institutions are facing – think, just to refer to recent years, of the financial crisis, the migration crisis, the rise of populism, the growing political and ideological polarization, the issues raised by multiculturalism, or the pandemic crisis. By definition, an emerging phenomenon presents itself with traits of novelty; consequently, studying it from an exclusively bottom-up perspective, in terms of the accumulation of empirical data, requires much time and costs, which hinders the ability to offer prompt and appropriate responses to frontier problems and issues. In addition, exclusively bottom-up approaches to new problems run the risk of not fostering the development of innovative interpretations, particularly when an in-depth understanding of phenomena requires going beyond their factual meaning, established in common sense. For example, an exclusively empirical approach would not have allowed the multiple manifestations of the political-institutional crisis of Western societies to be interpreted as a single process – the affectivization of the public sphere (Salvatore, De Luca Picione, et al., 2022). This is because, at the factual level, these manifestations are extremely differentiated from each other, lacking mutual connection.

Thirdly, the unified foundation of intervention promotes the consolidation of the social image of psychology. A unified image means less risk that, especially in inter- and multidisciplinary contexts, psychologists will be represented in a nonspecific way (think, in this sense, of psychologists working in educational communities, marketing, training, or organizational consulting). More generally, a unified image of the psychological profession operates as a driver for the enhancement of the profession, with its interpretive and intervention proposals, particularly in emerging fields (Cordella & Salvatore, 2021).

Of note, what has just been observed was already highlighted, in its political guise, three decades ago by Alan Kazdin (2008) in his role as President of the American Psychological Association.

> Insufficiently discussed is the importance of the unification of psychologists. Our scientific advances depend on increased specialization, broad collaborations and interdisciplinary networks. Yet, to keep our specialties robust requires that we bring to bear the discipline and profession acting as a unified whole on a daily basis. This facet of the unification of psychology is critical as we make the case to the public and policy-makers of what might make a difference (e.g., in health care and reimbursement of services, funds for basic research). Here, acting as fractionated or narrow special interests is not as adaptive as it is in making the substantive advances of our field. When it comes to making strong cases, partnering with other national and international organizations, and achieving goals that will concretely help our subspecialty interests, the heft of a large professional organization presenting a unified front, with experts in moving legislation, accumulated know-how, and contacts that can make things happen are for the good of individual segments of the field. It is stunning to see APA teams form on multiple specific and specialized interests (e.g., in research, education, practice) and respond to issues of public as well as professional importance. This aspect of APA is very much like an immune system that must hover and be ready to respond quickly to needs as they emerge from different sources. The unification of psychology is not incompatible with fragmentation and specialization. Indeed, unification is our protection that recognition of and resources for our many segments and areas of specialization are enduring and secure.
>
> *(www.apa.org/monitor/2008/03/pc)*

3 Scientific knowledge and professional action in psychology

The approach to psychological intervention proposed in this volume is based on a dialectical conception of the relationship between scientific knowledge and professional practice. We believe it is useful to precede the discussion of psychological intervention that we will develop in the following chapters with a brief discussion of this conception. More particularly, there are two aspects that we intend to examine: the active role of professional practice in the construction of scientific knowledge and the epistemic nature of intervention.

Historically, the relationship between science and the profession has been seen in psychology from an applicative perspective: it was assumed that scientific knowledge is produced in the research sites and then transferred and implemented in the context of professional action. Consider, for example, psychotherapy. There is widespread agreement in this field that the evaluation of different forms of intervention requires the use of the experimental paradigm (Randomized Clinical Trials, RCTs). Now, as far as our interest here is concerned, in order to ensure the methodological validity of the results, RCTs can only operate on simplified, decontextualized, and standardized forms of psychotherapy and, as such, are not representative of the actual modalities and conditions of the clinical action. For example, generally, patients characterized by comorbid conditions – namely, the vast majority of patients – are excluded by RCTs in order to estimate the effect of treatment on individual diagnostic categories reliably (Westen et al., 2004; see also Grasso & Stampa, 2011). Ultimately, in one of the most representative and historically fruitful areas of clinical research, the prevailing idea – and consequent practice – is that scientific knowledge is first produced under controlled laboratory conditions (RCTs) and *subsequently* applied to real-world intervention settings.

The applicative logic is still prevalent in the field of psychology; however, in recent years, a circular view of the relationship between knowledge and practice has gradually become more and more widespread. According to this conception, *knowledge is at the service of intervention* (Carli & Paniccia, 1999; Cordella et al., 2022) and because of this, it develops as a response to the epistemic challenges raised by problems posed by the users of the psychological function. According to this point of view, professional action is not only the place where psychological knowledge is exercised; it is also, above all, *production factor* of that knowledge. Indeed, it is in the context and because of professional action that many of the phenomena of psychological interest emerge and become defined, and in this way, they can be made the object of scientific investigation.

Professional action challenges scientific research in a plurality of ways.

In the most obvious terms, the profession systematically identifies emerging themes and issues in social and institutional contexts that demand to be interpreted and addressed, and in so doing, the professional system conveys the *social demand for knowledge* that greatly influences the scientific research agenda. It only takes even a cursory glance at the historical evolution of psychological research topics in different fields to grasp how it undeniably reflects the trajectory of social and institutional dynamics – the socio-cognitive impact of uncertainty, attitudes toward migration, perceptions of climate change, conspiracy beliefs, tele-education settings and devices, identity dynamics in the LGTB+ population, no-vax beliefs and attitudes are some of the very many examples of areas of research activated in response to issues and problems that have challenged psychology on both epistemic and practical levels.

More subtly, professional contexts of the use of scientific knowledge challenge the latter because they make the criterion of *appropriateness* cogent. This criterion operates in two distinct and converging ways. On the one hand, heuristically, the appropriateness of knowledge lies in the fact that it finds meaning and value as a resource that empowers professional action and, through the latter, end users. This means that the ability of theories to map phenomena effectively is a necessary but not sufficient condition of validity. From the point of view of professional action, scientific knowledge must organize the representation of the phenomenon in such a way that this representation favors the intervention, highlighting the factors on which to intervene, the processes that can regulate it, and conditions that can foster its evolution. For example, consider an interpretive model of school dropout that uses macro-social and structural indicators (e.g., unemployment rates, parents' education level, spatial distribution of users) as explanatory variables (for the sake of the example, we assume that such a model is empirically validated). Well, such a model would be appropriate if it framed the intervention addressed to actors who can act on macro-social and structural factors (e.g., public decision makers); on the other hand, it would not be appropriate, and it may even fuel a sense of powerlessness, if it were used in the context of an intervention aimed at an educational institution. This is for the obvious reason that it would offer no indication of what the actors in that school can do with the resources at their disposal to counter the phenomenon. On the other hand, appropriateness concerns the reflexive nature of social action. Indeed, according to this important point of view, it should be noted that, as a rule, psychological interventions are aimed at subjects (individual and collective). In other words, users of the psychological function are not empty vessels that the psychologist fills with scientific knowledge. Rather, users have desires, expectations, beliefs, implicit theories, attitudes, preferences, and interests – in a word, they are imbued with subjectivity. It is, therefore, illusory to think that the normativity of scientific knowledge governs the subjectivity of intervention contexts – people, as well as institutions and social systems, do not stop feeling, thinking, and acting in the ways they identify with simply because scientific evidence has sanctioned that a different way is preferable to them and/or more consistent with data. If that were the case, just to give a few examples, there would be no smokers, no gamblers, no no-vaxers, and we probably would not be so far down the road to environmental catastrophe.

This means that from the point of view of professional action, scientific knowledge is appropriate to the extent to which it solicits/promotes/supports users' reflective action – namely, the ability to revise and develop their way of operating *from within the action*. Consider the doctor-patient relationship. Vast amounts of research have highlighted the relevance, not only to the quality of the relationship but also to the effectiveness of health care treatment, of factors related to the physician's ability to listen to and recognize/take charge of the patient's emotional components. To use this enormous amount of scientific knowledge in a normative way – that is, to translate it into a set of "evidence-based" directions on how the physician should behave in order to increase patient cooperation – is to make poor use of such an asset. The physician – as well as any person imbued with subjectivity – will not change an ingrained attitude, of which he often does not even have full awareness and ability to regulate, because someone from the outside shows him that it is not functional. This is true regardless of the scientific soundness of the advice. He can change his attitude if he is helped to recognize the meaning of his own way of operating, to grasp its adaptive function and, at the same time, its costs, to explore alternative modes, etc. In a word, if the psychologist does not presume to export his knowledge normatively but sees it appropriately as a resource to foster and support the process of development of the physician's relational competence.

Finally, we recall a further challenge that the profession poses to scientific research: the urge to enhance the explanatory capacity and computational depth of interpretive models. In this regard, it should be noted that in many cases, psychological theories offer explanations of phenomena in terms of covariations between variables. For example, through a series of experiments, it has been shown that exposure to stimuli that evoke one's own death leads subjects to, among other things, embrace polarized beliefs and intensify identification with the in-group (Greenberg & Arndt, 2012). Following Marr (1982; see also Salvatore et al., 2021), we call this level of explanation *functional*. A functional explanation is one that answers *why* there is a certain phenomenon by identifying the antecedents that determine its occurrence. Of course, the functional explanation can go deeper, identifying factors (proximal causes) that mediate the relationship between the distal cause and its effect; however, it remains a model focused on interactions between discrete variables. Now, the point of interest here is that functional explanations express a potential for intervention that, though broad, is limited. They, in fact, by definition, can only ground interventions focusing on (distal and/or proximal) antecedents of the phenomenon of interest to be manipulated: if phenomenon A is caused by B, then changing B makes A change as a result. For example, research has shown that trust in institutions is the factor that most affects the propensity to vaccinate against COVID-19 (Cordella et al., 2023; Graffigna, 2021). On this basis, an intervention to promote adherence to the vaccination campaign (A) should aim to increase trust in institutions (B).

However, the functional explanation is not always sufficient, or it may lend itself to further development. These are the cases where cause-focused interventions are not feasible or, at any rate, are capable of producing limited impacts only. Indeed, in many circumstances, antecedents are difficult to isolate and modify, and/or are in large numbers, and/or are intertwined with each other, not infrequently weakly linked to the phenomenon of interest. An example of such a circumstance is psychotherapy – we know that it is effective; we also know many causal factors (e.g., therapeutic alliance, patient motivation, therapist competence, and personality) that foster this effectiveness (e.g., Orlinsky et al., 2004). However, these factors are hard to isolate, in some cases are difficult to modify, and, most importantly, operate in an intertwined, rather than linear, manner. Another example is offered by community dynamics. Research in community psychology has shown, for example, that the level of civism is influenced by perceptions of the quality of services and the level of community sense of belonging (e.g., Mannarini et al., 2019); however, such causal links are in some ways circular, rather than unidirectional; moreover, they are significant but limited in magnitude. Finally, returning to the earlier example of the causal link between trust in institutions and adherence to the COVID-19 vaccine – it is difficult to think that promoting adherence can feasibly be accomplished within the time frame required by the pandemic emergency.

In cases of the type recalled previously, it becomes relevant to complement the functional explanation with a model of the underlying process. We refer to this level as a *computational* explanation. At this level, the "why" is not about finding the antecedent but about modeling the mechanism that makes a certain cause bring about a certain effect (under certain conditions). Ultimately, if functional explanation connects input and output, computational explanation opens the black box within which the process that connects input and output takes place. Now, it is in the context of professional action, because of the need to enhance the capacity for effectiveness, that the limitation of functional explanation becomes apparent. From this point of view, professional action does not merely ask research for knowledge; its propulsive function is to qualify an epistemic standard – computational explanation – that actually broadens the horizons of the scientific enterprise, particularly in that central area of psychology represented by the theory of the change (Salvatore, 2021a; see Chapter 3).

Intervention as practical knowledge

In this section, we explore the dialectical link between scientific knowledge and professional practice from a complementary point of view based on the recognition of the *epistemic nature of professional action*. In psychological intervention, more generally in any occupational activity, professionals do not simply use knowledge defined elsewhere; rather, they elaborate, more or less implicitly and procedurally, a way of interpreting, employing, modulating, and sometimes redefining such knowledge because of the contingencies of the contexts of intervention. Even a superficial observation of the behavior and discourses of professionals engaged in their activities is enough to show how extensive the informal and implicit regulation of practices is, in contrast to the role played by formalized norms and procedures.

Above all, what can be grasped is how essential such a form of practical knowledge is in governing the extreme variability and dynamism of the context of relationships where such professionals work. Consider, for example, a psychometric instrument. Technical knowledge of the instrument (e.g., knowledge of its psychometric characteristics, mode of deployment, coding procedures, interpretation of results) is obviously a necessary condition for using it; however, it is not sufficient. The professional will have to make several decisions due to contextual contingencies that, in most cases, are not covered by the standardized and simplified form that technical knowledge around the instrument usually takes. For example, the professional may find themselves having to use the instrument under precarious logistical conditions or having limited time available; again, they may find themselves grappling with a user that, for cultural reasons, shows difficulties in understanding the meaning of items, as well as having to represent the results in a way that makes them usable by professionals of other kinds. In all these circumstances, and in a variety of others, technical knowledge of the instrument is not enough – it is supplemented by practical contextual knowledge that the professional constructs in the course of action as a way of adapting their action to the variable constraints induced by the institutional, organizational, and material conditions in which it takes place.

The practical and contextual knowledge that is produced from within the intervention does not concern only the conditions of use of the tools but the very way in which scientific knowledge and techniques are exercised, as well as their purposes. This last observation refers to the considerations made earlier about the criterion of appropriateness. More generally, scientific knowledge of a phenomenon does not include directions on how to use it successfully. The use of such knowledge is organized by the context in which it is exploited, the strategies and preferences of the actors involved, the type of problem posed, and the constraints and resources available. According to a complementary point of view, the same techniques only partly apply invariantly, according to their internal rules. In fact, in many circumstances, the *how* of the procedure is influenced by *why* and *for whom* it is used. The emblematic example of this is the interview – no matter how much one may codify it ex-ante, the conduct of an interview is a two-way dance that depends largely on the idiosyncratic purposes and manner of the participants (Paniccia & Salvatore, 1998).

The previously mentioned observation leads to the conclusion that the practical knowledge that makes up professional action should ultimately not be considered a source of distortion, an antagonist to the ability of technical and scientific knowledge to produce results. On the contrary, it should be recognized that scientific knowledge acquires intervention value only through, and in terms of, the practical and contextual knowledge of the professional. Moreover, it is precisely psychology that has highlighted the poietic character of professional practice (e.g., Zucchermaglio, 2002). Professional action is always exercised in the context and because of a community of practice – a dialogical field of negotiation of meanings that recursively nurtures the production and reworking of knowledge. Within that field, each professional actor deploys a repertoire of practical knowledge and implicit behavioral patterns, which are the expression of his or her own positioning within the distributed and informal network of expertise that substantiates every organized form of action (e.g., Valsiner & van der Veer, 2000).

The recognition of the epistemic and poietic nature of professional action has an important implication for the purposes of the discussion put forward here: if professional action is a form of implicit knowledge that grounds the very possibility of regulating the relationship between praxis and context, then scientific knowledge, rather than substituting for it, is called upon to enhance it, that is, its ability to substantiate competent forms of professional action.

Scientific research, then, is not called to "saturate" professional action with its knowledge. Rather, it has the strategic task of supporting the capacity of the psychological intervention to make locally produced knowledge available and usable, enabling it to make it explicit, validate, and systematize it. According to this point of view, scientific research stands as a dialectical interlocutor with respect to the practical knowledge exercised in the context of professional action. In other words, it is a set of methodological criteria, interpretive models, and theories that, on the one hand, constrain the forms of practical knowledge and, on the other, foster its explication and validation, thus its transformation into a shared asset. Ultimately, scientific knowledge has the function of promoting the *scientific-reflexive action of professionals:* scientific in the sense of being informed by scientifically grounded criteria and models; reflexive in the sense of being systematically oriented to recognize and revise the implicit forms of contextual knowledge that orient and at the same time constrain it.

Note

1 The expression echoes the title of Pirandello's novel, *One, no one and one hundred thousand* (English translation by W. Weaver) Marsilio, 1992 (Italian original version, 1926).

2
THEORY OF THE OBJECT

This chapter discusses the metatheoretical object at the foundation of the unification of the psychological intervention: the *dynamic of sensemaking* (hereafter, for brevity, also only: sensemaking). Our proposal is based on the cultural-semiotic psychology framework (Semiotic Cultural Psychology Theory, SCPT; Cremaschi et al., 2021; Salvatore, 2013, 2016c, 2018; Salvatore et al., 2021, 2022; Valsiner, 2007, 2014, 2020), which, by integrating cultural psychology and psychoanalysis (Salvatore & Zittoun, 2011; Salvatore & Freda, 2011), has elaborated a unique conception of the relationship between meaning, mind, subject, behavior, and society. We will use this theory to outline the terms of how the dynamic of sensemaking underlies subjectivity and the latter's recursive link with social life.

Needless to say, we do not consider our proposal of object to be the only feasible conceptual option; other general theoretical frameworks are possible, and a dialectic between different options would be desirable, as it would help to consolidate the paradigmatic foundation of the discipline and professional action. From this point of view, we believe that theories of object should aspire to be *exhaustive*, but without thereby expecting to be the only one. As models of fundamental dynamics, their theoretical validity lies in their ability to provide a foundation for the totality of psychological processes and their manifestations in the different spheres of life. Therein lies the exhaustiveness against which they are to be evaluated: the broader the class of phenomena that can be interpreted in terms of a given fundamental dynamics, the more valid the theory of that dynamic is. However, this does not mean that there must be a single fundamental theory. Fundamental theories are points of view, metatheoretical frameworks that interpret reality from a particular angle, highlighting some classes of relationships among elements, relegating others to the

DOI: 10.4324/9781003449362-3

background. Thus, general theories are not to be compared in terms of truth but in terms of heuristic capacity, i.e., according to the extent and depth of the interpretations they are able to ground. In this sense, no general theory needs to claim uniqueness to think of itself as the only one possible. On the contrary, pluralism among general theoretical models is desirable since dialectical confrontation among different options is the nourishment of the discipline's theoretical progress.

The chapter is divided into seven parts. The first section outlines the triadic theory of meaning that underlies the subsequent discussion. The second section delves into the characteristics of meaning that the triadic theory of meaning highlights. The third section aims to highlight, through the use of a plurality of examples, the multiplicity of phenomena that can be interpreted in terms of the dynamic of sensemaking. The fourth section outlines a conception of subjectivity as an emergent product of the dynamic of sensemaking. The fifth section delves into how meaning circularly links the individual mind and social activity. The sixth section offers a dynamic description of the circular link between sensemaking and social action discussed in the previous section. Finally, the issue of the specificity of the dynamic-semiotic model of sensemaking is briefly discussed in relation to the cognitivist conception of mind prevalent in psychology today.

1 What theory of meaning for psychology?

The centrality of meaning

The idea that meaning plays a central role in human affairs crosses a multiplicity of traditions of thought within the social sciences – from linguistics (e.g., Bühler, 1934/1990; Linell, 2009; see also Evans & Green, 2006) to sociology (e.g., Berger & Luckman, 1966; Zerubavel, 1999), from economics (e.g., Kahneman, 2003; World Bank, 2015; see also Salvatore, Forges Davanzati, et al., 2009) to organization theory (e.g., Weick, 1995), and from political science (Douglas & Wildavsky, 1982; Huntington, 2000) to anthropology (e.g., Douglas, 1986; Geertz, 1983) and psychoanalysis (e.g., Hoffman, 1998; Kirshner, 2010; Muller, 1996).

Recovering the Vygotskyian lesson, Bruner (1990; see also the special issue of *Integrative Psychological and Behavioral Science*, published in 2019) definitely helped psychology to recognize that cognitive processes are ways of attributing meaning to experience. That view, in its various nuances, now underlies many models of the functioning of the mind (Harré & Gillett, 1994; Salvatore, 2018; Valsiner, 2007, 2014, 2020), of communication and social behavior (De Rosa, 2013; Sammut et al., 2016), of learning processes (Cole, 1996; Iannaccone, 2010; see also Salvatore et al., 2003, 2005), of clinical (Carli & Paniccia, 1999), and cross-cultural (e.g. Heine, 2016) phenomena.

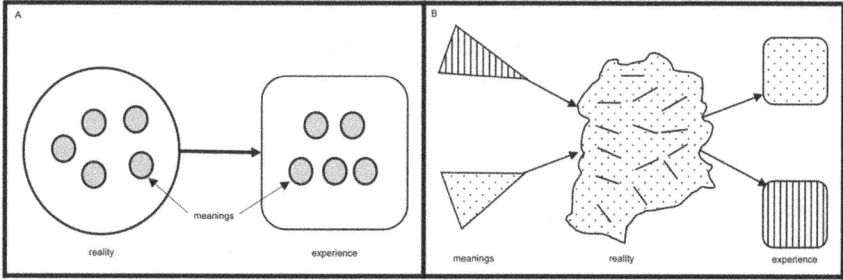

FIGURE 2.1   Two ways of considering the relationship between meaning and experience (A) Experience is the reflection of pre-existing meanings in reality. (B) Meaning is the way of making some elements of reality relevant, thus shaping them so that they emerge as contents of experience (adapted from Salvatore et al., 2018)

Meaning does not create reality; rather, it organizes the way humans interpret it, mediating the intra-psychological and communicative processes by which certain elements of experience are made relevant (Salvatore, De Luca Picione, et al., 2022), and related information is integrated (Peterson & Flanders, 2002). In doing so, meaning shapes the content of experience, of both the external environment and the internal world – the perception of one's own body and experiences.

Figure 2.1 depicts the constitutive function of meaning graphically: experience does not reproduce the objects of reality as they are given in the world (Figure 2.1A). On the contrary, meanings operate as polarizing lenses, filtering reality, selecting and thus giving stable form to some of its components, while the others are left in the background (Figure 2.1B; Bickhard, 2009; Manzotti, 2010).

The meaning of meaning

The meaning of meaning is far from obvious. Human beings live immersed in meaning and, for that very reason, do not recognize it. The prevailing conception of meaning in psychology is found in de Saussure's (1916/1977) dyadic theory of the sign. According to this theory, a sign is the union of a signifier/content and a signified/expression, with the latter standing for the former (Eco, 1975). According to this theory, meaning is the idea contained and conveyed by the sign.

This conception is consistent with the practical knowledge of common sense, which treats meaning as something that signs possess and convey. Whenever one assumes that meaning is an autonomous entity contained in/expressed by a word, image, or gesture – more generally, by a text – one is more or less implicitly referring to the de Saussurian view of meaning. However, copious literature has highlighted the many problems that arise when such a conception is used as the foundation of psychological theory (e.g., Gergen, 1999; Gillespie, 2010; Harré & Gillet, 1994; Lepper, 2012). We confine ourselves in what follows to highlighting two main criticisms (for a systematic discussion, see Salvatore, 2016c).

First, assuming that meaning is an autonomous entity, pre-existing the sign that conveys it, implies refraining from asking where it emerges from. In other words, the possibility of understanding the *intersubjective microgenesis of meaning* is lost, i.e., the dynamic of the relational field through which we experience signs as entities endowed with meaning. In doing so, psychology limits its focus of inquiry: it focuses on how the mind processes/manipulates signs as the vehicle of meaning, but it leaves in the background the fundamental question of how meaning emerges as a psychological reality – namely, the conceptualization of the dynamic that leads meanings to be constituted as the contents of subjective experience (De Luca Picione, 2021; Salvatore, 2012). To use an analogy, it is as if economics were limited to studying how banknotes are exchanged in the economic circuit without asking about the mechanism through which they acquire the capacity to convey economic value, that is, without asking how a piece of paper becomes currency and remains so over time.

Second, the idea that meaning is an independent entity that pre-exists sensemaking raises theoretical and methodological problems when it is intended to be adopted as an explanatory psychological construct. Indeed, from a theoretical-methodological point of view, meaning has no extensional properties – it is not a space-occupying element that exchanges energy/matter with other elements of the natural world. Therefore, treating it as having extensionality generates unresolvable questions: where is meaning? in the mind? in society? and if so, where exactly is it located? how does it move from one point to another in space? how is it possible for meaning, which is immaterial, to generate effects on the behavior of material organisms? Attempts to answer these questions have proved unproductive. The idea that meaning can cause behavior runs into two relevant conceptual problems (for a systematic discussion, see, among others, Fodor, 1983; Smedslund, 1988; for a philosophical analysis, see Wittgenstein, 1953/1958). On the one hand, it raises the homunculus paradox: if the semantic rule has explanatory power, this is possible insofar as it is interpreted in its own content, but this implies a further semantic rule guiding the interpretation of the first, which in turn requires a further interpretive rule, and so on ad infinitum (Salvatore 2016a, 2016b). On the other hand, the idea that semantic content is endowed with causal power displaces but does not solve the problem of identifying the psychological mechanisms that would allow the semantic rule to produce an effect on reality. For example, consider a person who, when asked how much three plus two makes, answers, "five." Now, the fact that the answer is the consistent outcome of the application of the addition rule is a necessary but not sufficient condition for explaining for what reason – namely, through what mental process the person implemented it (see in this regard Bickhard, 2009; for a similar critique, related to the problem of internalization of social representations, see Verheggen & Baerveldt, 2007).

An alternative. Peirce's triadic theory

According to the pragmatist perspective, meaning is the effect of the sign, the way the sign contributes to the regulation of action. Take a person who, upon entering the coffee shop, says to the barman – "a coffee, please," and receives a cup of the dark liquid. According to the pragmatist view, the meaning of the sentence consists of the barman's act of providing the person with the cup of coffee as the effect of the statement uttered.

Peirce offered a model of the semiotic dynamic underlying such an effect (Peirce, 1897/1932b; for a discussion, see Salvatore, 2016c). We quote one of the many definitions he gave of the sign:

> [the sign] . . . or *representamen*, is something which stands to somebody for something in some respect or capacity. It addresses somebody, that is, creates in the mind of that person an equivalent sign, or perhaps a more developed sign. The sign stands for something, its object. It stands for that object, not in all respects, but in reference to a sort of idea which I have sometimes called the ground of the representamen.
>
> *(Peirce, 1897/1932b, vol. 2, p. 228)*

According to the American philosopher, then, the meaning of a sign (the representamen; hereafter, sign A) is not "within" the sign; rather, sign A acquires its meaning by means of and in terms of the subsequent sign (hereafter, sign B), which sign A activates in the person's mind as a way of interpreting it. More specifically, the interpretation that sign B offers of sign A consists of defining the "respect or capacity" of the object that sign A represents – what Peirce calls *ground*. Sign A could stand for infinite aspects of the object; it is only through the next sign (sign B) that sign A becomes meaningful because it is representative of a particular aspect – among the infinite possible ones – of the object. For example, take a person who looks at a picture (sign A) of a landscape (object) and thinks (or states), "What a beautiful place!" (sign B). In this case, sign B is establishing that the *ground* of sign A is the aesthetic quality of the place. Imagine now that in looking at the picture, the person thinks, "How many beautiful memories!" In that case, sign B would establish as the *ground* of the picture the experiences the sense-maker has had in the past in the place in question.

The Peircean theory of sign is triadic, in that the sign takes on meaning because of the sign that follows – signifier and signified are not a pair: they come into relation with each other thanks to another sign (sign B). From a complementary point of view, it can be observed that the sign that follows implies the interpreter who produces it; this means that, differently from the Saussurian dyadic theory, meaning does not lie in the sign but is the product of the activity of the subject who interprets the sign: the *interpreter is constitutive of meaning*.

The triadic nature of the sign has several implications for psychology that deserve to be, albeit briefly, highlighted.

First, triadic theory implies an inversion of the relationship between meaning and sensemaking. Whereas in the dyadic conception, sensemaking is the mobilization of pre-existing meanings, in triadic theory, meaning emerges from the interpretive activity. It is worth pointing out that Peirce conceptualizes the process of emergence and its reproduction over time in terms of the maintenance of a relationship of correspondence.

> Namely, a sign is something, A, which brings something, B, its interpretant sign determined or created by it, into the same sort of correspondence with something, C, its object, as that in which itself stands to C.
>
> *(Peirce, 1902/1976, vol. 4, pp. 20–21)*

As mentioned in the previous section, the sign does not represent the object in all its qualities; rather, the sign defines a specific relationship with the object (called *ground*), and it is this relationship that is indicated and reproduced by the next sign: the relationship between sign A and object C is equivalent to the relationship between sign B and C, thus to the relationship between sign B' and C, between sign B" and C, and so on. Ultimately, this means that the sign never enters a direct relationship with the reality it represents – signs only relate to each other, not to the world they refer to. They are able to represent the world insofar as and by reason of the fact that they define relations among themselves that are assumed (by the interpreter) to be equivalent to the relation to the world. This ultimately means that the creation of meaning does not reflect and is not motivated by the characteristics of reality (of object C, according to the Peircean terminology recalled in the quotation); rather, it is the meaning – or rather, the chain of signs which sensemaking consists of – that makes the object emerge in the mind of the interpreter as something to be assumed as foundational and equivalent to the chain of signs that correspond to it. This leads to the recognition of the inherent temporality of meaning: the experience of reality emerges from the sequential combination of signs.

Second, triadic theory conveys a functional conception of the sign – a sign is any element of reality that takes on the function of standing for something else. In other words, a sign is not such by virtue of its inherent characteristics: anything can stand for something else and trigger a further sign. A relevant corollary of this functional definition is that not only ideas but also feelings, acts, affects, and, more generally, bodily states can operate as signs insofar as they enter the interpretive circuit. This conclusion is consistent with recent developments in the embodied conception of mind (Cuccio & Gallese, 2018; see also Salvatore, 2018; Salvatore et al., 2021).

Third, Peircean sign theory attributes a constitutive role to the interpreter. A sign is, by definition, addressed to someone. Sign B is the way the interpreter defines in what terms (i.e., in terms of what *ground*) sign A is meaningful to *her/him*. Triadic theory thus goes beyond the separation of *langue* and *parole* – meaning emerges from how signs are used.

2 Basic features of sensemaking

Triadic sign theory highlights some basic features of sensemaking that are relevant to psychological intervention.

First, sensemaking is *contingent*. As noted, meaning is not a pre-existing entity conveyed by the signifier but an *event*: the production of sign B by the interpreter, which occurs at a given moment, triggered by the chain of previous signs. In short, meaning is always and only "on-line": it is realized in the present moment (Stern, 2004) of its own emergence, and it needs to be continuously generated, like the balls that the juggler must continuously move to keep them suspended in the air. According to this approach, meaning is ultimately an abstraction: what actually exists is sensemaking – the continuous flow of signs; meaning is what happens with that flow in one of its infinite instants. To use an analogy, meaning is the instantaneous speed of sensemaking.

Second, sensemaking is *indexical*. According to Peirce, the sign interprets the previous chain of signs. This implies that meaning is constantly rewritten by the sign that follows – it emerges from how signs combine with each other in the contingency of the present moment. In short, the meaning of a sign is defined by the relationship the sign has with previous and subsequent signs. Therein lies its indexical nature: the context (i.e., the network of relationships between signs) is constitutive of the meaning of each of them (Salvatore, 2013). Note that indexicality is not only immediate: each sign can potentially rewrite the meaning of an entire sequence of signs backward. Humor shows such a capacity for retrospective impact: in various circumstances, what makes the joke funny is the fact that it forces the listener to redefine the meaning of the entire story previously told.

Third, sensemaking is *intersubjective*. Meaning emerges from how the sense-maker interprets the preceding sign. This means that the other – his/her interpretive activity – is constitutive of meaning and is part of the mechanism of its production. It is worth adding that the other can also be the same person who produced the previous sign. The otherness underlying meaning is structural: it lies in the idea, at the basis of the triadic theory, that the next sign (sign B) cannot merely "pick up" the meaning contained in the previous sign (sign A) but must necessarily rewrite it – in a word, interpret it. This introduces an inevitable hiatus between signs: the space for the exercise of otherness that at the same time allows meaning to be produced over time without at any time succeeding in establishing itself as given. If class conflict is the engine of history, otherness is the engine of subjectivity.

Fourth, sensemaking is *situated*. According to Peirce, any of the interpreter's responses can function as a sign insofar as it is, in turn, interpreted by the next sign. Any state of the subject – a feeling, a thought, a change in bodily state – can assume the function of sign, and this not as an outcome of the subject's will but as a consequence of being interpreted by the next sign and thereby made part of the semiotic chain. Ultimately, the situatedness of meaning lies in the fact that the subject is immersed in the semiotic flux – he does not choose to participate in it; on the contrary, his thoughts and acts – even those concerning intentions to regulate participation in communication – are intrinsically and inevitably a function of participation in the intersubjective field, i.e., in the generative semiotic flux of meaning that the subject mobilizes to make sense of their relationship with the world. This suggests the utility of making a distinction between *interpersonal* and *intersubjective* and using the first term to denote the phenomenal level of communicative exchange between people, reserving the second to refer to the theoretical construct that models the dynamic of sensemaking underlying any mental activity. According to this distinction, an individual may or may not find themselves in an interpersonal situation and can therefore choose whether to enter, remain, or leave. However, they are always, in any case, immersed in intersubjectivity insofar as the latter is constitutive of their mental activity, including that aimed at processing the decision of whether or not to participate in interpersonal contexts. The subject is inherently an intersubject.

Fifth, sensemaking is *embodied*. This feature complements the situated nature of meaning and extends its implications. Over the past two decades, the embodied view of mind proposed by Embodied Cognition has gradually become established (e.g., Barsalou, 1999, 2008; Gallagher, 2005; Lindblom, 2015). In brief, for what is relevant here, according to this view, the mind does not work on concepts encoded in symbolic units, which are structurally separate from perceptual and sensory input. On the contrary, concepts and representations are patterns of bodily activation made of the same sensorimotor substance as perception and movement. The subject does not have knowledge; it *is* knowledge (Baerveldt & Verheggen, 2012): knowing something does not consist of possessing a symbolic, abstract representation of the object; rather, it is a dynamic habitus, a propensity to (broadly speaking) relate to that object, which recruits the whole body (thus also the brain). Ultimately, to represent an object consists of simulating the interaction with it. Embodied Cognition, at least in its non-radical versions, does not deny that symbols can play a role in cognition; it asserts, however, that the symbolic dimension of mental processes is nonetheless rooted within and substantiated by the body, by the sensorimotor dynamic that constitutes the way in which the subject enters into a relationship with the world (Clark, 2005). This view is relevant because it allows us to move beyond the idea of meanings and, more generally, of cultural dynamics as abstract symbolic entities resting in a parallel Platonic world. Cultural meanings and dynamics are procedural propensities to act out the relation with the physical and social environment in a certain way – namely, they are pre-reflexive habits that substantiate the immanent form of the social action (Bourdieu, 1973/1977). Of course, cultural elements are encoded in symbolic representations (texts, images); ultimately, however, such representations gain meaning because of their grounding within the embodied mode of experiencing the world (e.g., Clark, 2005; for a systematic discussion of this view, in the context of the representation of inner states, see Barrett, 2006).

Finally, semiosis is *bivalent*. We noted previously that the interpretation provided by the following sign concerns the ground, that is, in what quality ("respect or capacity") the preceding sign stands for the object. From this, it follows that the sign has a dual valence. If the sign affirms something about a quality of the object, this ultimately means that it attributes a certain state of that quality to the object. At the same time, in doing so, the sign has defined the quality of the object it represents as the meaningful aspect to be represented; in other words, it has made a certain ground relevant in relation to the infinite other grounds in terms of which the object could be signified (Salvatore, De Luca Picione, et al., 2022). For example, in stating that the apple is red, two events are realized: on the one hand, one is pointing to red as the state of the chromatic quality of the object; at the same time, however, one is making color the relevant ground of the apple, neutralizing many other qualities of the object (taste, shape, cost, possession, function, etc.). The two events occur contemporarily, yet they are clearly not on the same plane: the characteristic of being red is attributable to the apple to the extent and on the condition that color is the relevant quality/ground. The pertinentization of the ground is thus superordinate to the attribution of the contingent state of the quality made pertinent. On the other hand, the pertinentization of the grounds does not occur prior to and independent of the attribution of its state. On the contrary, the two events occur simultaneously – by affirming a particular state of the quality, one is, at the same time, commensally, making the quality pertinent. The bivalence of meaning consists of this commensality: a sign indicates a certain state of affairs (the type of color) and in so doing defines the ground by reason of which the indication of the state of affairs acquires meaningfulness. It is worth adding that only the first operation is generally representable consciously by the subject. The pertinentization of the ground is an operation that remains outside of consciousness, carried out automatically: we are aware that we consider the apple red, but (unless someone points it out to us) not of the fact that by stating that the apple is red we have selected color as the relevant quality to be signified while backgrounding an infinite number of other potential grounds/qualities of the apple. One of us proposed referring to the two valences of the sign by the terms, respectively, of *Significance in Praesentia* (SIP) and *Significance in Absentia* (SIA) (Salvatore, 2016c). SIA is "in absentia" in the sense that it is not something that is said about the object; rather, it is the way it is constituted, thus the semiotic work from which the object arises, and which, therefore, allows us to talk about it.

The representation of sensemaking

Having outlined the conception of sensemaking, it becomes important to define the levels on which it becomes representable. In this regard, we propose distinguishing three foci of analysis: the *dynamic* of sensemaking, the *structure* that governs it, and the *content* it produces. This distinction is based on the reversal of meaning and sensemaking: if meaning emerges from sensemaking, then the understanding of meaning is not exhausted in the representation of its content; the modeling of the sensemaking dynamic from which the content emerges, and the organization (the structure) underlying it, also assumes importance.

The focus on the dynamic concerns how signs combine with each other over time and, in so doing, produce meaning. This focus is thus on the use of signs, on the individual and social processes – thinking, feeling, speaking, acting – that convey human interpretive activity, in brief, interactions. Ethnomethodology and discourse analysis are examples of this focus. A further example of analysis of the dynamic of sensemaking is provided by Salvatore et al. (2006/2009) in their analysis of the emergence of a shared frame of meaning between patient and therapist from within their communication. Specifically, the emergence of such a frame was described through the analysis of the evolution of the dimensionality of the communicative exchange between therapist and patient, indicative of the variability of the ways in which the two participants in the clinical exchange use words. The analysis showed that after an initial block of sessions, dimensionality underwent an abrupt decrease and then remained stable during the rest of the therapy; in other words, after an initial phase, the patient and therapist combined words in a less variable, more constrained way. The authors interpreted this result as indicative of the emergence of a shared frame of meaning, which organizes communication by making it more likely that certain words will follow a given word rather than others (e.g., that the phrase: "Good morning" is unlikely to be followed by, "How dare you?!").

Structure is another focus of meaning analysis. By structure, we refer to the organization of the dynamic of meaning, that is, the constraints that channel the selection of signs that enter the semiotic chain, analogous to how the riverbed defines the shape of its flow. Similarly to the case of wave spectrum analysis, the structure of sensemaking lends itself to being represented in terms of its decomposition into elementary components. Each elementary component describes one dimension of how the dynamic works, namely a part of the variability with which signs combine with each other (Salvatore & Venuleo, 2013). For example, the alternative representations of |migrant as threat| and |migrant as a person to help| can be decomposed into two bipolar dimensions of meaning: a dimension of evaluation (*good* vs. *bad*) and a dimension of power (*powerful* vs. *weak*). More specifically, the first representation is obtained from the combination of the *bad* and *powerful* poles, the second from the combination of the *good* and *weak* poles – being a threat means being bad and endowed with the power to harm; being a person to help implies being good – therefore deserving of help – and in need – therefore weak. The analysis of the cultural milieu of Western societies conducted by Salvatore and colleagues (2019a) is an example of a study of the structure of the dynamic of sensemaking. Based on responses to a questionnaire applied to representative samples of the populations of several European countries, processed through multidimensional analysis procedures, the authors identified some generalized dimensions of sensemaking – which they called *lines of semiotic force* – underlying the cultural milieu of the European societies investigated. We recall in what follows the description of the first two dimensions, to which we will also refer later (Chapter 3, Section 3.3.1).

Line of semiotic force 1. Affective connotation of the world: friend versus foe.
. . .
[This line of semiotic force] polarizes two opposite generalized, affect-laden ways of connoting the field of experience as a whole. On the one hand a positive connotation that qualifies the world as a fine, trustworthy object, that can be engaged with; on the other hand, a negative connotation qualifying it as unfair, meaningless, unreliable.
. . .
Line of semiotic force 2. Direction of desire: passivity versus engagement.

[This] line of semiotic force [consists] of what we propose to consider the direction of desire, namely the position assumed with regard the world: passivity versus engagement. Passivity is characterized by the sense of dependency on institutions, agencies and the primary network, thanks to which the subject can cope with the uncertain world; Engagement is characterized by the sense of agency, fostered by trust in people and institutions. In the final analysis, this line of semiotic force concerns the meaning of the world as the source of the action directed towards the subject (i.e., passivity) or, in contrast, as the goal of the subject's investment (i.e., engagement). In other words, being the object or the subject of desire (investment, commitment, acting on).

(pp. 61–65)

It is worth adding that structure and dynamic are circularly linked: the structure organizes the dynamic, and the dynamic in its unfolding reproduces – sometimes modifying it – the structure. From this point of view, the structure can be interpreted as the memory of the dynamic – the constraint that the past combination of signs places on the ways subsequent signs may combine. A path in the forest exemplifies the circular link between structure and dynamic – the path (the structure) is the effect of the previous paths performed (the dynamics). Each path contributes to shaping the trail, and this increases the probability that the next time the path will be "selected" again, in a recursive circuit that makes it more probable that what happens will happen again.

Finally, the third focus is on the content produced by sensemaking – meaning. A great deal of the attention that psychology gives to the phenomena of sensemaking concerns this focus. Many concepts are used in psychology to denote the content of sensemaking; some of them refer to meaning within people's heads – e.g., mental models (Johnson-Laird, 1983), fantasies (e.g., Klein, 1967); others refer to meaning that is active in the social context – e.g., social representations (Moscovici, 1961/1976), ideologies (van Dijk, 1998), worldviews (Koltko-Rivera, 2004), core values (Schwartz, 2016), and political cultures (Gamson, 1988). Although different from each other, these and other constructs share reference to meaning as content.

3 Meaning and sensemaking as the object of psychology

In this section, we anticipate some insights related to the semiotic interpretation of phenomena, that is, to their conceptualization as manifestations of the dynamic of sensemaking and/or meanings emerging from it. We do so in relation to the three levels on which psychological intervention can unfold – individual/micro-social, meso- and macro-social. We intend to highlight the ability of the psycho-semiotic theory discussed in this Chapter to operate as a unified object of psychology. We will take up some of these insights in Chapter 6.

Individual and interpersonal relationships

Several models have advanced semiotic interpretations of phenomena of clinical interest. For example, Venuleo and colleagues (Marinaci et al., 2021; Venuleo et al., 2018) have developed and empirically validated a reading of gambling as a function of specific patterns of affective meaning that character-izes the way gamblers make sense of the world (see also Salvatore, 2019a). In particular, it has been observed that, compared to non-pathological gamblers and non-gamblers, pathological gamblers are characterized by a strongly nega-tive view of the social context, perceived as anomic and unreliable.

Models from different traditions converge in recognizing the centrality of meaning in clinical intervention, particularly in psychotherapy. Constructiv-ist approaches (e.g., McNamee & Gergen, 1992), narratological approaches (e.g., Angus & McLeod, 2004), and dialogical approaches (e.g., Hermans & Hermans, 1995), as well as psychoanalysis, particularly Kleinian-Bionian (e.g., Ferro, 2005), intersubjective (e.g., Stolorow et al., 2001) and Lacanian (e.g., Kirshner, 2010) approaches, have delineated clinical exchange as a process of negotiation of meaning, which produces innovative meanings that can in turn influence the individual minds of participants (for a review, see B. D. Stern, 2013a, 2013b).

Local social contexts

The recognition of the centrality of meaning underlies several organizational theories. For example, organizational constructivism (Weick, 1995) views organizational behavior as an expression of how organizational actors make sense of their work context and the larger environment in which it is situ-ated. This view has been explored further by authors who have emphasized the role of organizational cultures (Schein, 1999; Zucchermaglio, 2002) and, more generally, of the forms and devices (e.g., rituals, ceremonies, sagas) of meaning-making that substantiate the life of organizations (Gagliardi, 1986).

From different points of view, in some cases converging (e.g., Salvatore et al., 2003), cultural psychology and psychoanalysis have proposed semi-otic readings of educational contexts. Cultural psychology, particularly that influenced by Vygotsky's work, has explored in depth the processes of co-construction of meaning that mediate learning processes (e.g., Cole, 1996; Perret-Clermont et al., 2004), the assimilation of implicit rules of participa-tion in educational contexts (Iannaccone & Ghodbane, 2005), the regulation of the exchange between teacher and learner (Pontecorvo, 1990; Venuleo et al., 2007), and the use of technologies (Ligorio, 2002). Authors drawing on the psychoanalytic tradition have conceptualized and empirically analyzed the role of school organizational cultures as matrices of meaning that organize the way institutional contexts and role functions are interpreted (e.g., Guidi, Fini, et al., 2015; Guidi, Venuleo, et al., 2015; Rochira et al., 2015). More recently, Venuleo et al. (2016) showed how dropout at the end of the second academic year can be predicted by the implicit meanings with which students organize the college placement experience at enrolment. Finally, Mossi and colleagues (2019) used the semiotic approach as the basis for constructing a school user satisfaction survey questionnaire aimed at analyzing the structures of latent meaning underlying the way students' families represent their relationship with school.

Community bonding has also been conceptualized and studied as a function of the dynamic of sensemaking. A key concept in this regard is the *psychological sense of community* (hereafter: PSoC), understood as the perception of the ability of the community to which one belongs to meet the needs of its members (e.g., Nowell & Boyd, 2014). PSoC is thus a semiotic construct – a belief through which people make sense of – and consequently regulate – their relationship with the social group with which they identify (for a review, see Albanesi et al., 2021). Several studies have shown that PSoC is inscribed in broader networks of cultural meanings – symbolic universes (Salvatore, Mannarini, et al., 2019) and core values (Mannarini et al., 2019) – in which the subject is immersed.

Macro-social contexts

Since the late 1970s, the social sciences have rediscovered meaning, recovering theories and analyses developed in the first decades of the 20th century by cultural anthropologists (e.g., Benedict, 1935; Boas, 1911; Mead, 1928), linguists (e.g., Bühler, 1934/1990; Sapir, 1921), and sociologists (Banfield, 1958). The so-called *cultural turn* cut across the different fields of social thought. In the context of sociological thought, cognitive sociology introduced the notion of *communities of thought* (Zerubavel, 1999, p. 9), highlighting that ways of perceiving, feeling, thinking, and acting are channeled by "cognitive traditions" rooted within the culture of the social group. At the intersection of economics, political science, and sociology, the various models that draw on the construct of social capital (Coleman, 1988; Putnam, 2000; see also Swendsen & Swendsen, 2009) have placed the sociocultural factor of *trust* at the center of the understanding of social and political behavior – and more generally the quality of functioning of political institutions. More recently, within this line of thought, the deterioration of trust in political institutions has been interpreted as a key factor in the progressive loss of legitimacy of the democratic system (Foa & Mounk, 2016). From a different but complementary point of view, political scientist Inglehart (1971; Inglehart & Welzel, 2005) has argued that the economic growth that has characterized Western democracies since the 1960s has led to a profound change in shared values, with the emergence of post-materialist values, which have operated as factors in the consolidation of liberal democracies. More recently, this interpretive framework has been developed further to interpret the political crisis of democratic institutions and the success of populist-authoritarian parties (Elchardus & Spruyt, 2016; Inglehart & Norris, 2017; Kriesi, 2014; see also Russo et al., 2020). According to this thesis, these phenomena are the precipitate of cultural motivations triggered by the growing inequality and insecurity generated by globalization.

The role of meaning in political life has also been highlighted on another level. In fact, several authors have pointed out that in established democratic countries, political conflict has lost the traditional class differences and the related issues associated with the social distribution of resources as its main reference, to be exercised today in reference to cultural and value differences (e.g., Scharfbilling et al., 2021; for an analysis related to the Italian context, see Schwartz et al. (2010) and Andreassi et al. (2023)). Finally, it is worth mentioning the interest that policy analyses express in the role played by emotions and identities, two additional concepts related to the dynamic of sensemaking (Hochschild, 2016).

The centrality of sensemaking has also been recognized in economics, the area of the social sciences where the alternative postulate of rational decision-making is most deeply rooted (see Salvatore, Forges Davanzati, et al., 2009). Two texts are emblematic in this respect. In 2000, Harrison and Huntington published a collection of essays, significantly titled *Culture matters*, focusing on the role of culture in countries' economic development processes. Despite no minor divergences, all contributions collected in the volume pointed out that the system of values and attitudes that characterized a given society is an essential component in explaining the differing capacity, even with equal starting conditions, with which different countries were able to pursue economic and social development. A recent World Bank report (World Bank, 2015) offered a systematic review of studies that have analyzed empirically how socio-cognitive processes influence economic decisions and behavior.

As we have already pointed out, meaning has also assumed centrality in various fields of psychology that deal with social and institutional phenomena. Models such as the theory of social representations (Moscovici, 1961/1976), social identity theory (Tajfel & Turner, 1986), the various forms of cultural psychology (e.g., Berry et al., 2002; Ratner, 2008; Valsiner, 2007), Terror Management Theory (Greenberg & Arndt, 2012), and Core Value Theory (Schwartz, 2016) each offer ways of conceptualizing the circular nexus that links shared interpretations of social and institutional contexts, social behaviors, and the material conditions within which actors enact interpretations and actions. In this general context, a range of recent research carried out on the basis of the psychoanalytic-culturalist model referred to in this volume has highlighted how the generalized worldviews with which social actors identify themselves influence a plurality of socio-cognitive processes – e.g., the choice between Leave and Remain in the Brexit referendum (Veltri et al., 2019), voting behavior (Mannarini, Veltri, et al., 2020) attitudes toward foreigners (Salvatore, Mannarini, et al., 2019), and attitudes toward vaccination (Rochira et al., 2019; Cordella et al., 2023). Finally, Madeo and colleagues (2021) showed that introducing cultural variables into a mathematical model describing the evolution of cooperation within populations decisively increases the model's ability to predict the evolution of cooperation within natural social contexts.

4 Meaning and subjectivity

In this section, we aim to highlight the role that the dynamic of sensemaking plays in shaping subjective experience. Our intent is to highlight how sensemaking provides vital substance to the sense of self and of being in relation to the world. We will discuss three aspects, which, in a convergent way, help in understanding the psychological significance of the dynamic of sensemaking: its constitutive role in experience, its role in nurturing the life value of representations, and its affective foundation.

The constitution of the content of experience

Common sense leads us to assume that feeling and thinking have an attributive function: they are ways we attribute (emotional, functional, semantic) properties to the mental representation of objects in the physical and social environment. However, in order to attribute a property to a given representation, that representation must first be constituted in the subject's mind. It is this process that we refer to with the expression *constitution of the contents of experience* (hereafter, for brevity: the constitution of experience).

Although on the fringes of contemporary psychology, we believe that the issue of the constitution of experience is of considerable importance, both from the theoretical point of view and, for what it is of interest here, from the standpoint of intervention. Indeed, the constitutive function of sensemaking makes this dynamic the foundation and nourishment of subjectivity.

Recognition of the constitutive nature of sensemaking is based on a long philosophical and psychological tradition (Kant, Husserl, Gestalt Theory) that has led to the recognition that the contents of experience (images, faces, landscapes, events, feelings, etc.) are not primitive elements but emerge from basic mental processes that organize sensory input into meaningful forms for the individual. According to this tradition of thought, reality is not made up of discrete objects and qualities; rather, it is a dynamic flow of energy-matter that operates as a global and continuous field of stimulation for the individual immersed within it (Manzotti, 2010). Consequently, the interpretation of experience is not just the process of attributing properties to already existing objects (e.g., the apple is red = attributing the property of being red to the apple) and mapping the relationships between them (e.g., the apple is on the table = the apple and the table are related by the above/below relationship). Before that, *signifying is the process by which the contents of experience are constituted, namely, they are "extracted" from the stream of variations as sufficiently stable forms and therefore perceived as content of the experience.* Qualities and relations can only be attributed once these forms have been extracted and thus constituted as contents of experience. Subjectivity is the way we shape the world before being the way we attribute properties to that shape.

Incidentally, it is worth noting that to claim that sensemaking is constitutive is not the same as embracing an idealistic view, according to which the mind *creates* its own experience, such that reality exists insofar as it is thought. As noted previously, reality exists independently of the subject, as a flow of energy-matter, and one cannot but assume that this flow has its own intrinsic organization, which places constraints on the creation of meaning (Fronterotta et al., 2018). Reality offers infinite possibilities for extraction, albeit limited – not all extractions are possible. Therein lies the difference between constituting and creating: sensemaking constitutes experience in that it shapes reality but still does so in one of the ways that reality allows.

Let us see in what terms the constitution of experience is the foundation of subjectivity. Let us start from what has already been noted previously: the constitution of a mental representation always involves the selection of a set of aspects (the ground, in Peirce's terminology) and the placing in the background of a – considerably larger – share of other aspects. Interpreting is, in this respect, similar to the work of the sculptor, who extracts a form by eliminating the rest of the material. Gestalt theory, and even earlier, Kant, taught us that, on a basic level, selection/extraction follows invariant transcendental rules. However, selection reflects human variability too: seeing the glass half-full or half-empty, a set of trees or the forest, the banknote or the piece of paper, are different ways of shaping objects, each of which represents an act of subjectivity – that is: the exercise of an option that inscribes the subject's imprint on experience.

From the point of view of intervention, the recognition of the constitutive – and not merely attributive – role of sensemaking enhances the psychological reading of phenomena and envisions a line of expansion of the professional action. In brief, conceiving the dynamic of sensemaking in a constitutive key offers the possibility of interpreting psychological phenomena at their root: in the way content is constituted rather than downstream of that dynamic – namely, when it is associated with attributes. Consider, for example, the vaccination campaign. Many people have shaped that domain of life in individual, concrete terms, figuring the vaccine as a medical device addressing the individual and relegating the political, institutional, and systemic aspects of the vaccine campaign to the background. It is worth noting that, according to the thesis we are discussing here, these people do not choose among alternatives all present in their domain of experience – for these people, the vaccine campaign is made experiential *through* and *in terms* of the selected form: for them, the vaccine campaign is the vaccine to be inoculated. Once experienced in this way, the subject will be able to access a vast but limited set of relevant features attributable to the object represented. The feelings, experiences, thoughts, speech, and behaviors of such persons will thus move within the framework defined by that set – for example, for such persons, the issue of the iatrogenicity of the drug will be cognitively and emotionally central, or the data regarding its efficacy, etc. Other characteristics, on the other hand, will not be subjectively relevant – for example, those related to the institutional and systemic dimensions of the campaign, such as the impact on healthcare facilities, the overall rationale for preventive measures, the international distribution of vaccines, etc.

The signs' value of life

From a complementary point of view, sensemaking is the source of subjectivity because the vital sense of being in relation to the world depends on it. Experience is lived as a self-evident mirror of reality: the contents of our mind are immediately assumed to be representative of the objects of reality to which they refer. As I run to get to the station, the representation of the train and its imminent departure for me are not mere internal representations; in absolute self-evidence, they are a fact of the reality, the-world-as-it-is.

Thus, internal representations have subjective cogency: they are endowed with *value of life*, according to the expression used by one of us (Salvatore, 2012). There are representations as having value of life that substantiate subjectivity: they enliven passions, fuel motivations, drive action, and give existential color to experience. Nations, money, institutions such as the municipality, marriage, and the soccer league, as well as objects such as plates, cutlery, screwdrivers, and so on, are not entities endowed with a life of their own, and that as such, our minds assume within themselves; rather, they are meanings that give reality a certain shape, so automatically and stably that they are experienced as if they were pieces of reality (Salvatore, 2016c) in a kind of ubiquitous Stroop effect.

Now, both theory and experience offer insights to recognize that such a Stroop effect is not a condition given a priori; rather, it should be considered the product of sensemaking.

From a theoretical standpoint, triadic sign theory leads one to recognize the inherent and unresolvable hiatus between semiosis and the world. The mind relates to the world (to the *dynamic object*, in Peirce's terminology) only through and in terms of the ground, that is, the property for which the sign stands. Moreover, as discussed earlier (see Section 2), meaning is not contained in the sign but depends on the relation between the current sign and the preceding and following signs. The sign, then, does not contain the thing to which it refers: the sign's capacity to stand for the thing must be constantly activated, moment by moment in the semiotic chain, through the continuous process of backward interpretation that the subsequent sign exerts on the representamen. This point is crucial to understanding subjectivity: the subject is never able to grasp reality in itself – the subject is locked into the semiotic flow, and from within, it can only use the next sign to keep alive the sense of being in relation to the world (see in this regard the analogy with the juggler used previously).

Experience, in this case, assists theory. We do not always experience mental representations as charged with the value of life in daily life. Generally, those who invoke Lady Luck do not feel that they are addressing an entity that actually exists. In many cases, it is the representation itself that may or may not take on the value of life, depending on the circumstances. Think of what happens at the cinema: we are immersed in the images that flow on the screen – for us, they are not just images; they are the living experience of a piece of reality in which we are participating. We suffer, we worry, we are moved, and we get angry with the characters, experiencing them as real entities. However, if the film's script is weak, or if disturbing events – the neighbor's chatting – intervene, the value of life effect fades away; as someone who knows about cinema said: emotion is interrupted. On the other hand, what happens to us when we find ourselves with a rude person for a neighbor at the cinema – or when we have made a bad choice of movie – is a ubiquitous process. From this point of view, many problems related to collective participation in the preservation of the commons (first and foremost, the problem of climate change) can be interpreted as an expression of the fact that for a significant portion of society, the representation of these goods possesses a weak value of life (Cremaschi et al., 2021). All this leads to one conclusion: if the value of life of representations is variable – between and within individuals, due to circumstances – then it means that it is the product of a particular psychological mechanism that deserves to be understood, as it underlies the subjective sense of being in relationship with reality.

The semiotic nature of affects

Triadic sign theory implies the interpretation of affects from a semiotic perspective. Consistent with Peirce's assertions (Poggiani, 2012), affects can be conceived as types of signs: signs consisting of patterns of bodily activation (Salvatore, De Luca Picione, et al., 2022). To the extent that the sign is an interpreter's response to the preceding sign, the affect is a sign insofar as it is a neurophysiological response that interprets in terms of its own basic hedonic value (e.g., in pleasant/unpleasant terms) and the state of affairs that triggered it (Salvatore & Zittoun, 2011; Salvatore, 2016c). Incidentally, this view is consistent with the Embodied Cognition thesis that any form of meaning is embodied – that is, consists of sensorimotor patterns that recruit the same neural systems involved in perception and movement (e.g., Barrett & Lindquist, 2008; Barsalou, 1999, 2008; Borghi et al., 2017; Cuccio & Gallese, 2018; Gallagher, 2005).

The pattern of bodily activation that substantiates the affective sign provides an interpretation of the entire domain of experience as one totality; more specifically, affects are global, hyper-generalized, and homogenizing signs (Salvatore & Freda, 2011). The activation pattern recruits the entire body-mind system (therein lies its global nature) and refers to the whole domain of experience (hyper-generalization), the latter connoted as a single entity to which the parts are assimilated (homogenization). For example, when a person is gripped by an affect of unpleasantness, this state does not merely connote the event/stimulus that provoked it but tends to radiate over the whole of the situation the person is experiencing. For affect, all cows are black in the dark night (or white in the bright day).

The global nature of affects explains their bipolar structure (Barrett & Russel, 1999; Osgood et al., 1957; Salgado & Clegg, 2011; Salvatore et al., 2017). Affects are not discrete individual categories but dimensions consisting of the juxtaposition of two opposing patterns of neurophysiological activation. For example, pleasantness and unpleasantness are not two different affects, but the two polarities of the same affective dimension. A central point of the semiotic perspective proposed here is that each affective dimension corresponds to a bimodal variation of a basic component of the relation to the world. In other words, each affective dimension is a bodily map of a "slice" of the entire variability of the relationship with the world (Salvatore, De Luca Picione, et al., 2022; for a similar view, see Stern, 1985). For example, the pleasant/unpleasant dimension maps the component of the self-world relationship consisting of the bimodal variation between a world that produces pleasure and a world that produces displeasure. The affective active/passive dimension (Osgood et al., 1975) maps the component of the self-world relationship consisting of the bimodal variation between the self that moves toward the world and makes it the target of its own activation and the self, which is addressed by the world's movement.

This view of affective dimensions as embodied maps of the components of the intersubjective landscape can be better understood if we refer to the early stage of the child-caregiver relationship (Schore, 2001; Trevarthen, 1998; Trevarthen & Aitken, 2001; Tronick, 2007; Tronick & Beeghly, 2011). At that stage, the infant's body produces global states of affective activation, each in response to the relational environment. For example, consider a mother holding her infant, seeking and holding his gaze, responding to his smile, and at the same time rhythmically cradling him, responding to the infant's vocalizations with progressive pitch intensity. It is plausible that such a relational environment activates an affective state of pleasantness in the infant as a response. Now, it should be kept in mind that the relational environment the infant experiences is inscribed in biological and cultural scripts; consequently, the dynamic qualities of such an environment tend to co-vary in a redundant manner. This causes certain covariations of these qualities to coalesce into specific patterns so that they are constituted into relatively stable components of the relational environment (e.g., the component represented by maternal attunement under conditions of low dyad activation). In turn, this allows the infant to consolidate over time an associative link between each relational component and the affective dimension (e.g., pleasant/unpleasant) associated with it. Over time, as the relational environment becomes more complex, its components will combine into sufficiently stable patterns, hereafter: *relational scenarios*. These scenarios will be experienced by the child in terms of a configuration combining the polarities of affective dimensions, each associated with one of the components of the relational scenario. For example, the affective configuration of arousing pleasantness recalled in the previous example is given by the combination of the pleasant polarity of the pleasant/unpleasant dimension and the arousing polarity of the aroused/relaxed polarity. In this way, the child will gradually form and consolidate in memory a series of affective activation configurations, each consisting of a combination of affective dimension polarities and operating as a map of a relational scenario. In the following, we will refer to such configurations of affective activation as *affective self-other schemas* (sometimes, for brevity: self-other schema) to highlight the function of interpreting the experience they perform.

Progressively, the affective self-other schemas are consolidated as sensorimotor memory patterns of the original relational world (Seganti, 1998), thus becoming the foundation of the interpretation of experience: when the adult individual is exposed to contextual clues assimilated to a sufficiently large number of features of a given original relational scenario, the corresponding affective schema is activated; in this way, the person re-experiences in the present the bodily state associated with the original relational scenario. Let us return to the example of the mother with the child in her arms. When the subject, once an adult, feel themselves being sought in their own gaze, or when they feel that the interlocutor is responding to their relational initiative, at the same time relaunching it, these perceptions may be sufficient to activate the self-other schema of excited pleasantness in terms of which, as a child, they experienced the relational scenario described. This is where the semiotic nature of affect lies: *every affect is an embodied sign that stands for a relational scenario experienced in the early stages of life*. Affect, however, is a special sign: it does not merely stand for the past experience of the relational scenario; affect actualizes that experience in the present moment. In other words, affect does not merely represent the bodily experience of the past relationship; it *presentifies* it. Remembering a painful incident does not make one feel pain;

activating the affective memory of an original painful relational scenario does. The homogenizing function of affects merges present, past, and future into one totality, embodied by the affective state of the body (Salvatore, De Luca Picione, et al., 2022).

Affective semiosis and subjectivity

The idea that underlying the interpretation of experience there are affective self-other patterns that reflect early relational experiences harks back to one of the central contributions of psychoanalytic theory: the idea that affective, unconscious patterns of meaning that emerge from the generalization of early relational experiences are at the grounds of mental processes (e.g., Bowlby, 1969; Klein, 1967; Stern, 1985) and shape the experience of the object – for example, the persecutory object, the nurturing object, and so on.

Reference to triadic sign theory allows this view to be complemented by the recognition of the function that affects serve in giving subjective substance to experience. From such a perspective, a self-other schema can be conceptualized as a basic ground, embodied in nature, by reason of which the subject makes sense of the present moment of relation to the world, mapping it in terms of a state of the body that stands for an original relational scenario. In what follows, we will refer to this level of human interpretive activity as *affective semiosis*.

As understood here – that is, as a constant monitoring of the relational meaning of the present moment – affective semiosis is ubiquitous: it is exercised continuously and systematically, intertwining with other levels of sense-making, offering them the embodied interpretive background of the relational scenario of which they (the other levels) are part. We refer in this regard to Barret (2006), who describes affects as a kind of physiological barometer through which the subject monitors moment by moment the state of the relationship with the environment.

Thus, affective semiosis does not act episodically, breaking in at some moments and remaining silent at others; on the contrary, it is *commensal* to the other levels of interpretive activity, those that follow the rules of logic. This means that the dynamic of sensemaking unfolds through a matryoshka mechanism: the sequence of signs *simultaneously* activates a plurality of grounds, of different degrees of abstraction, nested within one another. Let us look at an example. Take the coordinator of a working group who introduces the periodic team meeting, saying, "Colleagues, today we have a demanding job to do. The case to be investigated is particularly challenging; I am sure it will give us satisfaction." This statement conveys an operational meaning – it is a descriptive representation of the work program, of its quality of being demanding and challenging; at the same time, the statement is a form of affective semiosis, which conveys the relational scenario of being strong before the object mounting the attack (the challenging task).

It is the commensality of affective semiosis to the more general dynamic of sensemaking that makes the former the subjective substance of the latter: ultimately, *affects are the bodily memory of the relational experience of early life whose activation fills the signs mobilized in the present of the dynamic of sensemaking with vital meaning – with the value of life* (for a discussion of affects as the source of the life value of signs, see Salvatore, De Luca Picione, et al., 2022).

The interpretation of affect as the ground has another important implication, which points back to the constitutive role of meaning discussed in the previous parts of this section. Affect is not an emotional predicate that is attributed to a pre-existing content of experience; in fact, the ground is not the state of the quality that is attributed to the object but the quality that makes it possible for a certain state of the quality to be attributed. Picking up on what is discussed previously, the ground is the color, not the red: it only makes sense to say that the apple is red insofar as the ground made pertinent is the color. The same can be said of affect: being angry with a person is not simply the operation of attributing to the person the quality of being frustrating and deserving attack; rather, this feeling (the affect comprising it) is the way of giving pertinence to the relational ground/scenario whose state can be represented, among other things, as generating anger in the subject. This means that the other is presented in the mind through and in terms of its deserving to be attacked: for the subject, the other exists in the form of the target of attack; to use an image, affect is the cast that allows the form to be extracted from the liquid matter of the real (Salvatore & Zittoun, 2011).

It is worth adding that the bimodal structure of affect plays a central role in the mechanism underlying the constitutive power of affect outlined previously. The affective ground is not a discrete and/or one-dimensional quality (such as color, economic value, position in space, etc.). The bimodal nature of affect means that affective ground is a dimension of variability defined by two juxtaposed polarities. This means that the relational scenario actualized in the present by the affective state encompasses both dimensions, the active one and the one juxtaposed to it (see in this regard the concept of *Significance in Absentia*, Section 2). Based on what has now been said, we can return to the previous example and specify it further: the ground is not the frustrating object; the ground is the relational scenario of |receiving from the other|. This scenario can assume states that can be traced, on the affective level, to the two polarities of gratification and frustration. Anger, from this point of view, in activating a polarity, makes the entire field of variability associated with it present, namely, the relational scenario of |receiving from the other|.

5 Mind and culture

The previous section focused on the intrapsychic dimension of sensemaking. In this section, we address the dimension of the link between the sense-maker's interpretative activity and that which takes place at the level of the system (i.e., the collective dynamic of sensemaking that feeds the premises of meaning at the basis of the social action). That mind and culture are connected is a fact of experience, even before the thesis was advanced by a multitude of models, as well as by entire disciplinary fields (anthropology, cultural psychology, cognitive sociology). However, the question remains open as to how mind and culture keep themselves interrelated. In what follows, we present how Semiotic-Cultural Psychology (SCPT) addresses this question. We will focus on two aspects: first, what the sharing of cultural meanings consists of, and second, how individuals internalize such shared meanings.

Culture as a field of variability

SCPT shares with many other theories the idea that the cognitive processes that substantiate sensemaking cannot be conceived as a function of mechanisms and rules contained in the individual's head. Cognition is situated within the social group, shaped by the needs and requirements of regulation of the social action. More specifically, the situatedness of mental activity lies in the fact that the interpretations based on which the subject experiences reality – how and what he or she feels, thinks and acts – are grounded, constrained and substantiated by the system of semiotic resources of the social group.

The SCPT adopts the term *cultural milieu* to denote the system of semiotic resources shared by the social group. However, the shared nature of the cultural milieu should not be interpreted in consensual terms, that is, as indicating that all members agree on the core meanings qualifying the group's culture. Indeed, it should be kept in mind that the system of semiotic resources is a network of signs linked by convergence and opposition relationships. What group members share are not single interpretations but the structure of relations among signs that gives meaning to such interpretations (the Significance in Absentia, see Section 2) (Markova, 2003; Salvatore et al., 2017). This means that embracing a certain meaning (e.g., holding a certain belief) means establishing differences from other meanings that are active within the cultural milieu (e.g., distancing oneself from a different belief, rejecting an opposing belief) (Salvatore, Valsiner, et al., 2019). In short, what group members share is the terrain on which they can differentiate and enter conflict with each other: *the culture is the space of negotiability of meaning.* Consider, for example, the discussion around anti-COVID vaccination. The conflict between those in favor and those against has reached highly polarized levels in many countries. This polarization, however, is fueled by a set of oppositions that must necessarily be shared by all participants in the conflict; in fact, taking a stand for one of the alternatives can sound meaningful only because of the alternative that is thereby denied (Salvatore et al., 2017) – for example, individual freedom vs. collective interest, collective resource vs. profit-making tool, and safe vs.

dangerous. Participation in shared culture thus does not lie in agreeing on a given meaning about the vaccine; rather, it lies in using the same oppositional structures. It is in this sense that the cultural milieu can be defined as the *space of variability of the social group's interpretive activity*; that is, the domain of differences within which different trajectories of sensemaking are representable by those who produce them as contingent forms of the participation itself. In short, the cultural milieu is the semiotic field that defines the possible movements of feelings, thoughts, and acts in a given society.

The affective foundation of the normativity of culture

Based on the conflictual interpretation of culture advanced previously, let us now address the second question: how are the signs active within the cultural milieu internalized so as to be able to exercise their normativity – that is, their capability to trigger, ground, and channel individual cognitive processes?

In short, the thesis of SCPT is that basic cultural meanings are affective in nature, and for this reason, *they operate simultaneously as semiotic resources of the cultural milieu and on the grounds of individual minds*. This means that, ultimately, individual cognitive activity and the social group are not two separate processes. On the contrary, they are produced based on the same fundamental system of semiotic resources offered by affective semiosis: affects are the natural *esperanto* that attunes individual sensemaking with that of others.

On the level of empirical analysis, SCPT has modeled the affective foundation of the cultural milieu through the construct of the *symbolic universe* (Salvatore et al., 2018). The conceptualization that SCPT proposes of symbolic universes is partially different from how this concept is generally used in social sciences (Berger & Luckman, 1966). According to the SCPT dynamic-semiotic conception, a symbolic universe is a system of pre-reflexive underlying assumptions, a *worldview* that substantiates a comprehensive interpretation of the subject's relationship with the worlds of social life. The worldview that the symbolic universe expresses is affective in nature – it is an embodied habit, a propensity to perform, in the different circumstances of social life, a certain dynamic pattern of feelings, thinking, and acting. Underlying symbolic universes are affective self-other schemas: each symbolic universe is a pre-reflexive belief about the world shaped by an affective schema (Salvatore, Valsiner, et al., 2019). The interpretations – feelings, opinions, attitudes, behaviors – that a symbolic universe channels and nurtures can also be largely different in their content; what holds them together and makes them an expression of a single, organic form of being-in-the-world is their affective valence. For example, a person may experience deep distrust of institutions, on the one hand, and feel immigrants as a threat, on the other: there is no logical connection between these two feelings and the beliefs/discourses they nurture; what makes them homogeneous, so that the person can feel they are an expression of a coherent point of view, is the negative and persecutory affective connotation of the context they express.

Three features of symbolic universes deserve to be recalled here as indicative of their affective nature. First, symbolic universes are holistic – each provides a connotation of the entire field of experience as a single totality. Second, symbolic universes are inherently relational; that is, they are ways of entering into a relationship with the world; in other words, a symbolic universe is not a description of/belief about a certain state of affairs; rather, it is a propensity to enter a relationship with the world in a certain way. For example, affectively connoting the world as "good" is a predisposition to act in terms of caring, being close, sharing, etc. Third, symbolic universes are not governed by the logic of justification: they do not use the true/false or right/wrong criterion; rather, they follow the affective logic of everyday thinking (Tonti & Salvatore, 2015). Because of this, each symbolic universe polarizes and brings to the fore those aspects of reality that are consistent with it, backgrounding the others; in doing so, it functions as a *premise of sense* that reproduces itself through the search for the elements that confirm it.

Given the oppositional structure of affects (cf. Section 1), each symbolic universe defines its own meaning because of its juxtaposition with other symbolic universes active within the cultural milieu. Salvatore and colleagues (2018) identified five symbolic universes active within the cultural milieu of a cluster of European societies (Cyprus, Denmark, Estonia, Greece, Italy, Malta, Netherlands, and the UK):

- *Ordered universe.* The world is a welcoming, beautiful place to inhabit. People, institutions, services, and the future deserve trust. What is right is also effective.
- *Interpersonal bonds.* Relationships with close people and the emotional experience such relationships provide are the only things that matter. Such experience makes life beautiful and satisfying.
- *Caring society.* Societies and institutions support people by providing the resources they need for their development. This nurtures full confidence in life, in the future, and in one's own agency.
- *Niche of belongingness.* The world is an inhospitable and threatening place. Pessimism, distrust, fatalism. The group one belongs to is the only shelter to survive.
- *Others' world.* Anomia, despair, fatalism. The world belongs to those with power. To the losers, all that is left is to live by the day and try to survive.

A subsequent analysis showed the structure of semiotic relations underlying the five symbolic universes – the *semiotic field* in the terminology adopted by the authors (Salvatore et al., 2019b). This structure was described in terms of three generalized dimensions of meaning, referred to as *lines of semiotic force* (see Section 2). For example, the *other's world* is contrasted with a *caring society* and *interpersonal bond* along the line of semiotic force *affective connotation of the world*, with the first symbolic universe placed on the *foe* polarity and the other two on the *friend* polarity. In turn, *caring society* is contrasted with *niche belongingness* along the line of semiotic force *direction of desire*, with the first symbolic universe placed on the *engagement* polarity and the second on the *passivity* polarity (see Figure 2.2). This means that the profound differences recorded at the level of the content of the symbolic universes are nonetheless recognizable as such due to the fact that they are juxtaposed positionings on dimensions of meaning (the lines of semiotic force) shared by all those embedded in the cultural milieu: on the one hand, the impact that social reality has on the subject, in the two affective configurations of friendly reality vs. enemy reality; on the other hand, the position taken towards reality – passivity (receiving from) vs. engagement (going toward). As can be seen, these two lines of semiotic force correspond to affective self-other patterns traceable as fundamental organizers of experience already in the early stages of life. Moreover, they correspond to two of the dimensions of affective meaning (evaluation and activity) that over the course of more than half a century, the endless literature around Semantic

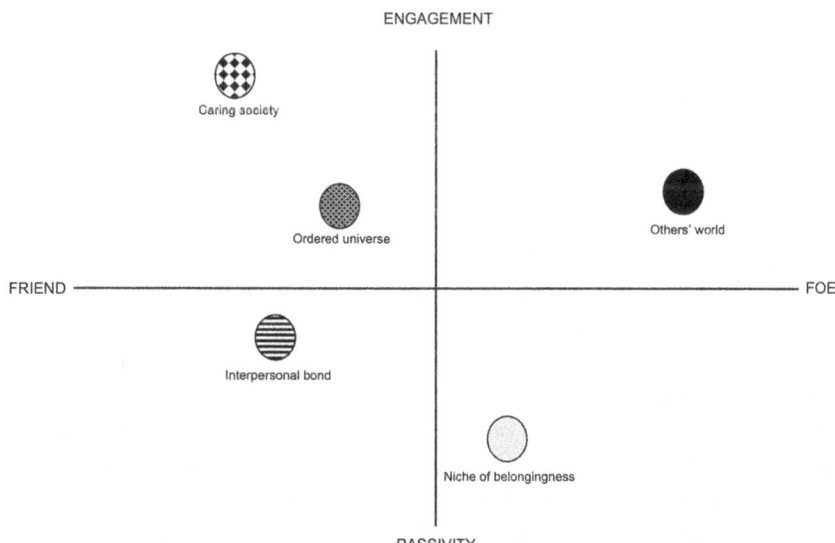

FIGURE 2.2 The semiotic field of the cultural milieu of European societies (defined by the first two lines of semiotic force) and the position of symbolic universes in it

Source: Adapted from Salvatore et al. (2019b, p. 74)

Differential has identified across a plurality of activity domains and cultural-historical contexts (Osgood et al., 1975).

The observations made so far should have clarified the thesis advanced by SCPT about the role of affects as the "glue" of mind and culture. In the final instance, SCPT does not answer the question of how cultural meanings are internalized and operate normatively in the individual mind. Instead, this theory offers a way of conceiving the relationship between mind and culture that enables such questions to be overcome. From the point of view of SCPT, in fact, the meanings active at the level of cultural milieu, or rather, the affective meanings underlying the cultural milieu (i.e., symbolic universes and lines of semiotic force), do not need to be internalized since, being universal forms, biologically grounded in the way the body functions, they are at the same time the basis of individual sensemaking. Consequently, such fundamental meanings organize the interpretive activity of all human beings (as we have noted, not in the sense that they determine their products, but in terms of defining oppositional structures that channel and constrain the variability of interpretations) and in so doing also define the semiotic field of the entire cultural milieu.

To use an analogy, sensemaking operates like a *jam session*: the musician follows his or her own individual interpretive line, which moves because of a universal structure of acoustic similarities and oppositions and is, for that reason, equivalent to that which organizes the performance of other musicians. The ensemble effect that is realized is thus the emergent product of the interaction of the movements of individual musicians, each nevertheless guided by the same acoustic semantics.

The hierarchical organization of semiotic resources

The cultural milieu is, of course, not only composed of symbolic universes – any culture provides the social group with a set of semiotic resources (Zittoun, 2006): beliefs, rituals, artifacts, symbols, relational scripts, values, etc. Such semiotic resources are the product of how social actors organize their mutual contingency within the contexts of social action. For example, an organizational ritual is a way of crystallizing a pattern of hierarchical relationships that characterizes the life of a given organization. This means that the elements of a culture are produced on the basis of – and thus within the constraints of – the symbolic universes at the foundation of the social action.

It follows that it is possible to prefigure a mapping of semiotic resources in terms of a multi-level typology, differentiated according to their degree of abstraction. Preliminarily, let us point out that, following a definition of this concept that can be traced back to Bühler (1934/1990; see also Salvatore & Valsiner, 2010), the term abstract here is used to denote the process of foregrounding/making relevant some aspects of what is represented and relegating the others to the background: the greater the abstraction, the narrower the set of features made relevant. A highly abstract set is thus a collection that adopts a low number of features as a classificatory function. For example, the category "living being" is more abstract than "human being" because the classificatory function of the former is poorer than that of the latter – fewer features are needed to define a living being than to define a human being.

Based on the definition now outlined, we distinguish five levels of meaning due to the degree of abstraction involved (for a similar approach, though used with a different analytical purpose, see Valsiner, 2007).

As implied by what has been said previously (see Section 1), at the highest level of abstraction there are the affective self-other schemas (for a view of affects in terms of high abstraction, see Borghi et al., 2017). At this level, meaning is a state of the body that can be associated with an infinite class of reality configurations and thus cannot be related to any specific empirical element.

We have already observed that symbolic universes (see Section 5.2) are the ways self-other affective schemas are actualized in the multifarious circumstances of social life. Each symbolic universe can thus be considered the *local* product of an affective schema. This is provided that we give the term "local" a broad meaning: the set of experiences that substantiate the subject's participation in the spheres of social life. We consider a symbolic universe a meaning at a lower level of abstraction than the self-world schema because, though generalized, a symbolic universe is representable by reference to (though global) features of the social reality and associated experience (Salvatore et al., 2018). The symbolic universe construct is obviously not alone in mapping cultural meaning at the level of high abstraction we are considering. For example, constructs such as core values (Schwartz, 2016) and the individualism-collectivism continuum (Trandis et al., 1988) refer to fundamental meanings that provide a comprehensive interpretation of social life. Following Valsiner (2007), we can call *hyper-generalized signs* the meanings placed on this level of abstraction.

Hyper-generalized signs enable the regulation of social action and, in so doing, the production of meanings that shape the interpretation of experience within specific domains of life. We define *generalized signs* as those meanings placed at this lower level of abstraction. Domain beliefs are a subclass of generalized signs: overarching interpretations of an entire domain of social life, which guide how we make sense of experience and, thus, how we feel and act within that domain. Examples of domain beliefs include a sense of community (e.g., Peterson et al., 2008), political values (e.g., Schwartz et al., 2010), and views of nature (Douglas & Wildavsky, 1982).

In turn, generalized signs organize the interpretation of the objects/events that populate the domains of life in which they are active. Thus, they ground the production of meanings related to the characteristics of such objects/events. This is the level of meanings concerning the *collections of discrete objects* (hereafter collections). Psychotherapy, vaccination, migrants, sports, and art are examples of collections as understood here. An example of interpretive activity referring to collections is involved in the many ways people relate to food. For some people, it is nourishment, for others, pleasure, for others, entertainment, for others, exploration, for others, temptation, etc. A similar discussion could apply to the way people approach pets, technological devices, music, and so on.

At the lowest level of abstraction, we find meanings referring to discrete objects, to *singularities*. Such meanings may relate to events ("The Italian national soccer team won the European championship in 2021"), people ("Sigmund Freud was born in Freiberg in 1856"), physical entities ("The sun follows an elliptical orbit around the sun"), social ideas ("My child's school adopts effective inclusion strategies"), and imagination ("Harry Potter was a student at Hogwarts School of Witchcraft and Wizardry"). The role of the embodied meaning referring to a singularity is evidenced by how our mode of relating changes, often in ways that are difficult to perceive, depending on the person with whom we are relating. With some friends, we are more prone than with others to physical contact, ironic banter, searching looks, etc.; this is not an intentional choice but a reflection of sensorimotor routines established over time into habits.

Before concluding, two caveats.

First, the hierarchy of abstraction levels that we have outlined previously should not be understood as a rigid classification but as a flexible ordering criterion: whether a certain meaning is to be considered a generalized or hypergeneralized sign, a singularity, or a collection depends on the context. What the proposed hierarchy enables us to point out is that whatever way the individual meaning is considered, it will still be possible to inscribe it in a hierarchy of levels of abstraction.

Second, the relationship between the levels of abstraction is circular: the levels influence each other both top-down and bottom-up. On the one hand, as already noted, more abstract semiotic resources channel and constrain the selection of less generalized signs. For example, people's political beliefs are influenced by their worldviews (Mannarini, Veltri, et al., 2020). On the other hand, the use of signs of lesser abstraction is how signs of greater abstraction reproduce themselves over time. And this brings us to the theme of the next section.

6 Meaning and social context

The previous section proposed that affective meaning is the foundation of the link between the mind and society. To this end, the discussion focused on the structural features of affective meanings (in particular, their generalized and prereflexive nature and their subjective valence). In this section, we complete the argument by highlighting the circular process between sensemaking and social action. To this end, we consider the two sides of the issue separately: first, the role that sensemaking plays in regulating social action, then, the way social action allows the sensemaking dynamic to be reproduced. This will allow us to conclude with the mutual inherence of sensemaking and social action.

The premises of sense. The semiotic nature of the regulation of social action

Let us begin by highlighting the role of sensemaking as a social regulator: meaning is the foundation of social action. Every social practice to be exercised needs a system of meanings that is taken for granted as an established premise of sense (e.g., Berger & Luckman, 1966; Douglas, 1986). The premise of sense reduces the potentially infinite variability in the actions of individual actors and, in so doing, enables the coordination of action.

The premise of sense does not define what is canonical; in excluding a space of potential variability, it also leaves in the realm of the possible what constitutes the thinkable violation of the canonical, one could say: the canonical deviations from the canonical. One thinks of the soccer player who is sent off by the referee because of a serious foul on an opponent; the foul is a canonical deviation – it is a violation of the norm, which nevertheless remains within the domain of the social action in question, within what the rules of the game envision as a deviation.

Even the most trivial social interaction would not be possible without a constraint being placed on the potentially infinite variability of individual action. For example, imagine a person meeting an old friend on the street and stopping to say hello. To be performed, even such a simple gesture requires that a very large class of potential acts of both participants in the interaction remain outside the options of the possible, relegated to the background of unthinkability: it is not part of what can be expected to happen that the acquaintance responds to the greeting with an insult or an assault, or that they roll on the ground, walk on their hands, violently hit their own face, take off their clothes, and so on. If the infinite possibilities of the interaction evolution were allowed, the person would not be able to predict the evolution of the interaction resulting from their act, thus remaining paralyzed.

Two aspects of the relationship between the premise of sense and social action deserve to be highlighted.

First, it is important to note that constraints on the variability of individual action operate outside their consciousness by definition; in other words, they are not representable contents but taken-for-granted assumptions or *institutions* (Harmon, 2020): areas of blindness that act in the background.

They define that which is unthinkable, which remains outside the realm of the possible. Actors do not have premises of sense; rather, they are immersed in them and exercise them as habits or prereflexive procedures (Bourdieu, 1973/1977) that shape their feelings, thoughts, and behaviors by imposing boundaries on their possible trajectories. Only from an external point of view, actionable by those who are not immersed in them, the premises of sense can become objects of representation.

It is worth pointing out that the unthinkability of the premise of sense and its instituted character is essential to enable it to perform the task of allowing actors to coordinate with each other. Indeed, the moment a premise of sense comes to be represented and enters discourse, it acquires the status of a declarative norm. Now, a declarative norm is a statement by which a set of alternatives is denied – for example, the obligation to pay taxes makes sense to the extent that there is not an alternative option to not pay them. Thus, one can understand that as soon as a premise of sense becomes representable, it also conveys the representability of its own violation, consequently opening a front for social negotiation. This means that the declarative norm paradoxically increases, rather than reduces, the variability of action, making social action less predictable and more uncertain. Consider, for example, the value of democracy. Until a few years ago, in Western societies, this value was not an object of representation – it was a premise of sense: discourses and actions inconsistent with it were unthinkable or, where they occurred, were perceived somehow as a scandal, an attack on the sanctity of the constituted order. Democracy, in other words, was not an object of the public discourse but its foundation – its premise of sense, indeed. Today, democracy is under discussion, and this is both the consequence and the cause of the fact that it has lost its valence of instituted premises, its foundational capacity, plunging into contingency: a meaning that, in the very act of being affirmed, implies and conveys the possibility of its negation, and therefore open to social negotiation.

Second, it should be emphasized that, as understood here, the concept of coordination does not refer to a functionalist view of the social order: coordination is not synonymous with cooperation, agreement, or integration. By coordination is meant the state of social action characterized by the fact that each actor possesses a representation of the possible evolutions of the other actors, thanks to which inferences can be made about the current and future state of the action. From this point of view, a group of people involved in a fistfight is an example of a highly coordinated action: each participant in the fistfight has a representation of the space of variability in the actions of other participants and can predict the evolution of this situation of social practice, and thus adjust their action accordingly. More generally, it could be said that social practices of conflict are those that exhibit the greatest degree of coordination – which other social practice can be carried out with greater coordination than fighting with a stranger, where actors have a high prediction of every contingency in the almost total absence of a shared knowledge base?

The performativity of meaning. The Matthew effect

As noted previously, premises of sense are outside the actors' representational field: they are habits, prereflexive propensities to activate certain sensorimotor patterns as a way of interacting with particular configurations of social action. They are, therefore, learned and reproduced in the way habits are formed and reproduced: *through repetition* – the more a sensorimotor pattern occurs, the more it is consolidated, that is, the greater the likelihood of repetition in the future (Salvatore, 2018). This ultimately means that the premises of the sense of social actions are not reproduced over time through negotiation; rather, they are reproduced (in some cases modified) by the performing of the action. The more redundant the form of social action, the more the premise of sense associated with it is consolidated.

Therein lies the *performativity* of meaning: in its very unfolding, social action reproduces the premise of sense that is immanent to it (for an empirical model of this process, see Salvatore et al., 2006/2009). For example, the literature has shown that several interpretations of the vaccine and the social context – primarily, distrust of public institutions (Cordella et al., 2023; Graffigna, 2021) – underly the rejection of COVID-19 vaccination. Thus, these studies show that meaning provides a foundation and directs action. However, there is also the opposite direction to consider: vaccination rejection is the acted-out – performative – mode through which the interpretations of context are exercised, and in this way, reproduced over time through the social practices they trigger – the no-vax discourses, the responses of institutions, and the forms of negotiation with pro-vaccination people (Rochira et al., 2019).

The performativity of meaning lends itself to be epitomized by what we propose to call the *Matthew effect*. In the Gospel of St. Matthew, it is reported that Jesus, after being resurrected, meets some disciples and tells them, "Where two or three are gathered together in my name, there I am" (Matt. 18:20). We find in this Gospel passage a powerful image of the intersubjective dynamic of performative reproduction of the premises of sense: a social action ("two or three will gather together") finds regulation through a shared intersubjective premise of sense ("in my name") and in so doing makes such a premise a fact ("there I am").

It is worth pointing out that social action does not merely reproduce premises; in doing so, it nurtures the *semiotic value* of signs, too, i.e., their ability to represent the objects of reality to which they refer stably (Salvatore et al., 2021). On the theoretical level, from the triadic model of a sign (see Section 2), it follows that the semiotic value of a sign consists of the distribution of other signs with which it relates: the more polarized this distribution is – i.e., the narrower the range of other signs with which it is associated – the more limited are the ways the sign can be interpreted, thus the greater the predictability, specificity, and stability of its meaning. On the level of experience, a sign with high semiotic value is one whose meaning is felt (and thus used) as self-evident by the interpreter, as if it were the immediate reflection of reality. Countries are examples of signs with very high semiotic value: meanings experienced and practiced as if they were facts and things of the world, no different from elements such as water, stars, and stones (Carrettero & Kriger, 2011). On the functional level, the semiotic value of a sign consists of its ability to reduce the actors' interpretive variability and, thus, to represent the objects of social action in ways consistent with the demands for its regulation. On the operating table, the semiotic value of the sign "scalpel" lies in its ability to compel the assistant to hand the surgeon exactly the instrument he expects to receive.

Now, the semiotic value of signs depends on the stability of the premise of sense. In fact, premises of sense determine the interpretive context of signs (the ground, according to Peirce's terminology); consequently, the greater the stability of the interpretive context, the more stably signs are interpreted. Think, for example, of how material elements such as cell phones, pens, and clothes show (in many cultural settings) a not very high semiotic value. They are signs whose meaning is unstable, as they are interpreted because of a plurality of interpretive frameworks: under certain circumstances and in the context of certain social practices localized in certain areas of society, they are interpreted by reason of their functional qualities; in other circumstances by reason of their aesthetic qualities, and in still others by reason of their quality of being drivers of identity (Klein, 1999). In contrast, consider sacred objects – they have very high semiotic value in that the interpretive framework that signifies them remains stable, to the extent that the religious textuality of such signs is experienced, even by many nonbelievers, as immanent to them.

We thus arrive at the conclusion that social action nurtures the semiotic value of signs insofar as, by its own exertion, it consolidates the premises of sense underlying the interpretative stability of signs. The more the action proceeds without perturbation, that is, keeping itself within the margins of the established premises of sense, the more the latter, like any other form of habit, are consolidated and, consequently, stabilize the semiotic value of signs involved in them.

Sensemaking and action

To simplify the exposition, in the previous two sections we treated the two directions of the relationship between sensemaking and action separately. However, what we have said should be sufficient to show the recursive connection between the two terms. The premises of sense ground the regulation of social action, which in turn, in its making, reproduces the premises of sense. To the extent that such a circuit operates without relevant perturbations, action and the premises of sense consolidate each other, and in so doing, they nurture the sense of self-evidence of the experience of social life: the premises of sense remains in the background, working as the instituted foundation of the thinkable, and social action takes the form of a predictable landscape, in which actors move by reason of a prereflexive map of its possible evolutions.

Money is a particularly illustrative example of the recursive link between premises of sense and action. Banknotes are pieces of paper, signs devoid of immanent meaning. The economic value they convey, that is, the interpretation of the piece of paper as a banknote, emerges from their use. Actors use this type of sign within a premise of sense that greatly constrains the variability of action. From the outside, we can describe this premise as the assumption that no other uses of the piece of paper are conceivable except those that imply that it has economic value. Thus, for example, it hardly ever happens that someone uses banknotes to paper the walls of their house (unless they do so as a way of displaying economic value or contempt for it; in such cases, the use would be internal to the premise of sense recalled previously). From the actors' internal perspective, such a premise of sense is not an object of representation – rather, it is a habitus consisting of a limited set of ways of using the piece of paper. As an effect of the stability of such a habitus, of its instituted character, the interpretation of the piece of paper as a banknote is consolidated to the point of being "fused" with the sign. The triadic valence of the sign collapses to the dual form in terms of which the sign is perceived at the level of common sense. In turn, the stability of the meaning |banknote| makes the piece of paper a powerful device for regulating action: every member of the social group knows the different ways in which banknotes regulate social action – from shopping to robbery, from making/receiving a loan to gambling. The social actions mediated by banknotes thus reproduce themselves effectively, and in so doing, they, in turn, convey and consolidate the premise of sense at their foundation. In this way, the pieces of paper to which we are referring constantly absorb semiotic value. Their economic meaning assumes the character of self-evidence, to the point that a socially determined Stroop effect is realized: people perceive banknotes, not pieces-of-paper-that-they-interpret-as-banknotes (Salvatore, 2012; see also the concept of inter-objectivity, Harré & Sammut, 2013). Economic meaning takes on the constitutive value of experience: it gives shape to experience, already at the perceptual level.

Before concluding this section, let us recall a point of eminent theoretical interest, which nevertheless deserves to be clarified both for reasons of systematicity and for its implications on the level of intervention. The discussion so far implicitly assumes that sensemaking and social action are two different dynamics that recursively interact with each other. To a first approximation, this assumption is useful at both heuristic and expository levels. However, a deeper analysis of the concepts leads one to recognize that sensemaking and social action are not distinguishable on the ontological level. They are the same fundamental dynamics, represented by two different points of view, and related languages. In other words, a *principle of identity* is being affirmed here: sensemaking and social action are related to each other, as are the movement of water molecules and the vortex they create; that is to say, they are the same dynamic represented at two different scales of observation.

The recognition of the embodied character of meaning leads to this conclusion. Indeed, if every sign is ultimately a pattern of sense-motor activation, then the chain of signs making up the dynamic of sensemaking is, at the same time, a chain of variations in the state of the sense-makers' bodies, i.e., a pattern of social action. Think of a discussion between two people – it is at the same time and commensally an exchange of signs and a social action, commensally in the sense that the same elements that substantiate the dynamic of sensemaking – the words, gestures, and movements produced – are those that substantiate the social action.

Ultimately, then, all regulation of social action is, at the same time, the intersubjective form of functioning of actors' minds (for a similar conception, see Lindblom, 2015).

7 An aside. Information and meaning

The idea that sensemaking is the fundamental dynamic underlying psychological phenomena does not contradict the cognitivist view of the human mind that underlies a great deal of contemporary psychology. SCPT moves within the same paradigmatic perimeter as cognitivism, especially in Embodied Cognition's reworking of it, where it recognizes as a fundamental object of investigation the way in which the human organism – the mind-body unit that is instantiated in action – mediates the relationship between stimulus and response.

Having said that, we believe that the dynamic-semiotic view presented in this chapter enriches and generalizes the cognitivist conception of the mind by valuing the subjective and social depth of cognitive processes (e.g., Salvatore, 2018; Valsiner, 2007). As we have said previously, SCPT interprets cognitive processes because they are the way human beings shape their being-in-the-world (Bruner, 1990; see also Grazzani & Brockmeier, 2019; Smorti & Fioretti, 2019; Salvatore, 2019b). In this sense, mental activity does not process information about the environment; rather, it shapes it, "filling" it with meaning endowed with a value of life (Salvatore, 2012; Valsiner, 2020). It is in this sense that the theoretical concept of sensemaking is to be understood as an extension of the notion of cognition: sensemaking implies but is not reduced to the operation of attributing semantic qualities to objects; it is the human activity through which the interpreter continually constitutes them-selves as a subject, by making experience something-that-has-sense-for-itself.

Several implications of this extension have been outlined throughout the chapter. First, the recognition of the central role that affective semiosis plays in mental activity as the foundation of subjectivity, interpretation of experience, and social action. Second, the consideration of the inherently performative and pragmatic nature of meaning: on the one hand, meaning is reproduced through the action it enables to regulate (performativity of meaning); on the other hand, affirming something is an act, through which social action is regu-lated (pragmatics of meaning). Third, the possibility of conceptualizing the mutual inherence of mind, culture, and social action in a unified way, thus recomposing the hiatus between the micro, meso, and macro levels of analysis, between mind in culture and culture in mind, to use a formula with a wide following.

It is these implications, with the expansion of interpretive potential they bring about, that motivate our proposal to consider the dynamic of sensemak-ing as the metatheoretical object underlying psychological intervention.

3
THEORY OF THE CHANGE

This chapter concerns the second component of GTPI: the theory of the change. This is central to the entire conceptual architecture we are outlining. The psychological intervention aims at promoting change – that is, at introducing a difference, at making a certain course of events and/or a certain set of characteristics take on different values than they otherwise would.

The chapter is divided into six sections. In the first, the general terms of the approach discussed in the chapter are introduced. In the second, this approach is clarified through comparison with the logic prevailing in contemporary psychology, which focuses on mapping empirical relationships between phenomena of interest and their antecedents. In the third, some reasons for the usefulness of the proposed model of change are discussed. The three questions that change theory proposes to answer are also presented: the patterns (*what*), the mechanism (*how*), and the catalyzers (*under what conditions*) of change. The fourth section presents a typology of semiotic changes based on the levels of abstraction discussed in the previous chapter. The fifth focuses on the mechanism that fuels change. The sixth discusses the conditions that determine how that mechanism operates.

1 Preliminary notes for an epistemology of change

A terminological premise

As a preliminary matter, two conceptual and terminological distinctions should be made.

First, it is useful to distinguish the level of phenomena from that of the dynamic underlying them. Unless one embraces a radically behaviorist

DOI: 10.4324/9781003449362-4

approach, the focus of psychology is the intervening dimension that mediates between environmental input and behavioral output: the "O" of the classic S-O-R schema. Occurrences at the level of the phenomenon – which we will refer to in what follows as *mutation* – therefore, need to be explained in terms of the (broadly speaking) latent psychological processes that produce them. Secondly, a distinction must be made between the change as such and the conditions that trigger and fuel it – hereafter: *catalyzers* – as well as between the catalyzers and the actions/devices that convey/activate them – hereafter: *vectors*.

Figure 3.1 describes the semantic space defined by the two distinctions proposed. The dynamic of sensemaking undergoes a change over time (indicated in the figure by the change from white to gray) as a result of conditions internal to it (catalyzers), activated by environmental factors operating at the level of reality (vectors). The intervening change will have a phenomenal manifestation, representable in the mutation of the state of affairs of interest to the intervention. For example, the socio-cognitive conflict theory (Doise et al., 1998) holds that in the condition of game interaction with a peer having a different perspective (vector), the socio-cognitive conflict thus generated (catalyzer) fuels the process of accommodation (change) and this results in increased performance effectiveness (mutation). The peers with different perspectives and performances are observable elements of the phenomenal reality; socio-cognitive conflict and accommodation process are theoretical constructs through which the latent intervening mechanism is represented.

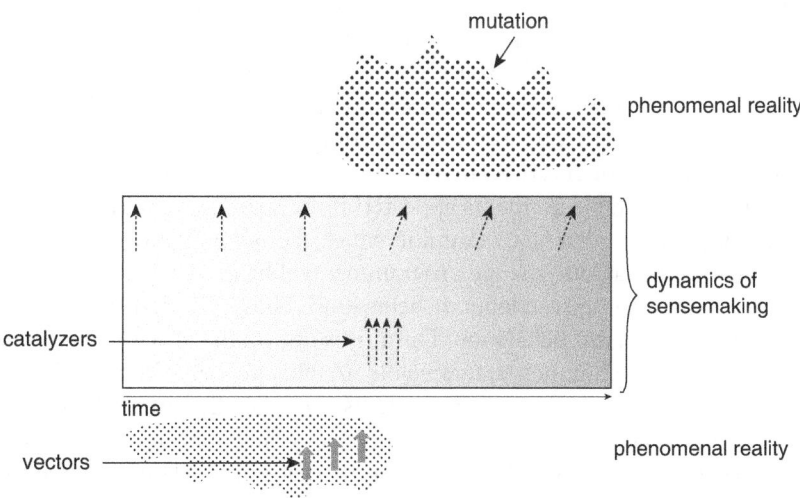

FIGURE 3.1   The components of the dynamic of change

On this basis, we can identify the three fundamental questions that the theory of the change that will be developed in this Chapter aims programmatically to answer:

- *what changes* – the variations of sensemaking that make up the change;
- *how does it change?* – the mechanism that generates the change;
- *under what conditions does it change?* – the catalyzers that activate that mechanism.

The issues of the vectors needed to activate the catalyzers and the modification in which the change of the dynamic results at the level of phenomenal reality are aspects that are covered by the theory of the action and the theory of the client, respectively (see Chapters 4 and 5).

Map of antecedents versus theory of the change

Most psychological research is aimed at explaining phenomena of interest through the identification of antecedents. One might, therefore, conclude – and this is generally the case – that antecedent mapping is the theory of the change underpinning psychological intervention: having identified the drivers that generate the problem or the factors associated with the desired outcome, the intervention has to act on such drivers and factors so that the problem is removed or the outcome achieved. What Dutch psychologists Steg and Rothengatter (2017) write in the introduction to a highly regarded handbook of applied social psychology is an effective formulation of this logic.

> First, in order to design effective solutions for social problems, we have to understand which behaviour causes the given problem. Applied scientists can best focus on behaviour that significantly contributes to a social problem and where interventions would have the most impact in resolving these problems. In our example, speeding by moped riders was studied because moped riders are relatively often involved in traffic accidents, while, in turn, these traffic accidents appeared to be strongly related to speeding. Second, it is important to examine which factors influence the particular behaviour. Behaviour-change programmes will be more effective when they target important antecedents of behaviour. Thus, we need to understand which factors cause behaviour. Third, it is important to understand which intervention techniques are available to change behaviour, taking into account which behavioural antecedents are typically targeted by various intervention techniques. In our example, speeding appeared to be strongly related to moped drivers' attitudes and social norms. Thus, interventions should best focus on changing attitudes and social norms related to speeding, for example, by designing information campaigns that stress the risks

associated with speeding, or emphasize that important others would disapprove of speeding.

(pp. 1, 3)

So, the theory of the change underpinning the intervention on the problem behavior – moped-riders' speeding – is based on mapping its antecedents (and selecting the most relevant and addressable ones) – attitudes and social norms of moped drivers – and consists of the idea that changing the latter has the effect of changing the former.

The theory of the change outlined in this volume follows a different logic. This logic does not deny the relevance of the empirical analysis of the factors associated with the problem and/or outcome being pursued. However, it considers it necessary to supplement such analysis with an understanding of how the dynamic of sensemaking must change for (a) certain antecedents to vary and (b), in turn, such modifications to produce the outcomes being pursued.

To stay with the example proposed by the Dutch psychologists, as understood here, the theory of the change would consider the detection of the link between moped-riders' tendency to exceed speed limits and their attitudes/social norms related to driving behavior the starting point from which to start in order to answer the following questions: what interpretation of the road traffic context underlies moped-riders' driving and their attitudes/social norms? What practices and discourses are fueled by and at the same time fuel this interpretation? What semiotic structures underlie this interpretation? Along what developmental trajectory can such structures evolve? What conditions can the interpretive activity of the actors involved (moped-riders, car drivers, control bodies, service providers, etc.) catalyze this development? The answer to these questions would enhance the intervention from two perspectives: on the one hand, it would provide an understanding of whether and to what extent moped-riders' behaviors and associated social attitudes/rules are expressions of – and thus are bound to – more general processes of sensemaking not immediately referable to the target behavior (speeding) – for example, the representation of motorcycling as an act of freedom, with respect to which the norm takes on persecutory significance. On the other hand, the answer to the questions would make it possible to identify the socio-communicative forms that optimize the possibility of perturbing the processes of sensemaking underlying the actions of moped-riders, thus fostering change in their attitudes, social norms, and associated behaviors.

In short, behaviors, attitudes, beliefs, and other phenomena of interest to psychology change if the underlying dynamic of sensemaking changes. The theory of the change is the part of the general theory of intervention that is concerned with modeling what it consists of, under what conditions, and how such change can occur.

One objection that might be raised at this point is that most psychological interventions do not adopt the approach we have proposed, but that does not mean they stop being effective, and therefore, this approach is not necessary and deserves to fall under the blows of Occam's razor. Our response to this objection is that, in fact, every psychological intervention is based on a theory of the change, i.e., on a belief about how human interpretive activity can vary. The question is whether such a theory is explicit and based on scientific parameters or is the common sense one implicitly available to members of the social group, thus also to psychologists. In terms of the example we are referring to, one may ask: is the hypothesis that motorcyclists' attitudes may change as a result of "information campaigns that stress the risks associated with speeding, or emphasize that important others would disapprove of speeding" based on a scientific model or is it an implicit, common-sense belief about the possible effects of certain types of communication? In other words, do we use practical knowledge derived from our membership of the social group or models developed by scientific psychology to formulate this kind of hypothesis?

The reader will know by now our answer to this question. However much scientific evidence we may accumulate demonstrating the effectiveness of a communication plan and, more generally, of an intervention technique/procedure, it may help us to clarify *whether* the intervention is effective, not *why*. In other words, the question of understanding the dynamic underlying the ability of the antecedent to produce its effect will remain open.

2 The black box

To prepare an answer that is model-based, not commonsensical, as to why and under what conditions the psychological intervention is effective is anything but simple. It involves opening the black box that links phenomena and antecedents. As we discussed in Chapter 2, sensemaking is a highly abstract metatheoretical concept; the theory that proposes to conceptualize how it varies over time cannot but be so as well. The opener needed to open the black box is, therefore, theory, or rather, a theory that guides the selection, interpretation, and use of empirical data. The mechanisms contained in the box are out of sight (otherwise, the box would be transparent or of another color, but still not black); since they cannot be observed directly, they must therefore be reconstructed abductively (on abduction, see Chapter 4, Section 3) on the basis of a solid theoretical framework. It can thus be understood how much of contemporary psychology, because of its empiricism (see Chapter 1), prefers to skirt around the box in search of the links between input and output rather than opening it up to plumb the mechanisms it contains.

Skirting around . . .

In this section, we present three examples of what we mean by the metaphor of skirting around the black box of mechanisms of change.

The first example is offered by what is happening in the field of the empirical study of psychotherapy. In this context, a growing number of studies – so-called process-outcome studies – aim at identifying factors associated with the outcome of psychotherapy (e.g., therapeutic alliance, patient motivation, therapist adherence to the clinical model). Such works do not attempt to provide a computational explanation of the psychotherapeutic process, i.e., to model the dynamic of change underlying it. Rather, they are aimed at detecting characteristics of the clinical exchange and the participants in it who, because of their covariation with outcomes, can be identified as factors of success (or failure) of treatments – they are analyses *in* the process, rather than *of* the process (Salvatore & Gennaro, 2015; Salvatore et al., 2010).

Socio-cognitive theories of uncertainty provide our second example. Although there are also significant differences in the way of defining the constructs used, the type of responses generated, and the causal mechanisms, most scholars working in this field agree that exposure to uncertainty induces individuals to adopt beliefs and/or behaviors that serve to cope with the disorienting impact of such exposure. For example, according to *Terror Management Theory* (TMT) (Greenberg & Arndt, 2012), when induced to represent their own death, people respond with a range of strategies, including adherence to polarized religious and/or political beliefs, in order to mitigate the anxiety that the thought of death triggers. The explanation for why this happens is that such strategies allow the person to intensify the bond of belonging so as to project themselves beyond death. Another example of such theories is the *Compensatory Control Theory* (Landau et al., 2015), according to which people are motivated to maintain a sense of controllability of the world and thus are inclined to adopt strategies to restore that sense where it is weakened. For example, experimental studies conducted in the context of this model have shown that people exposed to conditions of uncertainty related to loss of control tend to value institutions with control functions, as well as to express their belief in a normative God (but not in a God connoted in the key of love) with greater intensity. What we are interested in highlighting here is that this type of explanation focuses on the link between the antecedent (uncertainty) and its effect (subject responses). The causal mechanism that fosters this link remains in the black box. It is explained through a posteriori, functionalist reasoning: if a subject responds in a certain way, it is because of the function that this response serves to reduce the adverse impact of uncertainty. This sort of reasoning is based on at least three common-sense assumptions: 1) the individual is always motivated to avoid/eliminate the aversive valence of the experience of uncertainty; 2) the individual is able, even if implicitly and/or unconsciously, to manage the experience of uncertainty by identifying the response that allows them to counteract the aversive valence arising from uncertainty; and 3) the individual chooses the response because of the latter's functional ability to counteract the effect of uncertainty.

The preference for skirting around the black box rather than opening it is even more evident on the meso- and macro-social levels. See in this regard what North American community psychologist Jason (2013) writes in his book with the indicative title *Principles of Social Change*. The author recalls the work of an English physician, John Snow, who, in the mid-1800s, succeeded in stopping a cholera epidemic that had already claimed thousands of lives among the London population. At that time, the bacterial cause of cholera was not yet known – the epidemic was thought to be the effect of harmful properties of the air. Snow discovered that cholera cases were thickening near a public fountain; he therefore decided to turn it off, and by doing so, the contagions ceased. This result was thus achieved without a prior understanding of the mechanism of contagion. From here, the author derives a general principle:

> In short, although we will not always know the exact reasons for a social problem, we can still develop second-order change plans that successfully address the heart of the issue.
>
> *(p. 11)*

To put it in the terminology used in this paper, Jason's thesis is that in order to produce change, it is sufficient to identify an empirical association between the phenomenon of interest (cholera) and a factor that can be acted upon (the relationship between the location of the contagions and the fountain); varying the latter results in a modification of the former (on this, see also: de la Sablonnière, 2017).

. . . or opening it

The study of the therapeutic process offers examples of the opposite approach, too – namely, of the effort to open the black box. In this regard, one can refer to the theory of referential activity (Bucci, 1997). It models the therapeutic process on the basis of a general theory of cognitive functioning – the multiple code theory – which conceptualizes mental activity as operating according to three modalities – sub-symbolic, iconic, and verbal-symbolic. The three modalities are connected to each other through the referential process, by which sub-symbolic patterns are translated into images and words and vice versa. In this way, sensory experience is mentalized and made communicable. The referential process underlies the ability to regulate emotions and communicate them, as well as to understand other people's mental states. On this basis, psychopathology is conceptualized as a disarticulation of translation processes from one modality to another, and psychotherapy is modeled as a referential process with a cyclical pattern in which phases of sub-symbolic activation are followed by phases of iconic and verbal-symbolic translation, which in turn activate new sub-symbolic patterns. In psychotherapy, the therapist's referential activity supplants, supports, and feeds the patient's referential activity so that the patient can integrate levels of their own mental functioning progressively. As can be seen, the referential activity model does not focus on cause-and-effect linkages. Rather, it describes the overall way the process works, the dynamic underlying its unfolding over time. Referential activity is not an observable feature – it is a construct by which one enters the black box of the mechanisms that fuel the phenomenal reality.

The *Maintenance Meaning Model* (MMM) (Proulx & Inzlicht, 2012) differs from many of the uncertainty theories in its attempt to open the black box. This model focuses on the psychological process underlying how people react to conditions of uncertainty. Authors assume that uncertainty causes a destabilization of the meaning system with which the individual is identified; in turn, destabilization triggers an aversive physiological activation of alarm to which the individual reacts with a palliative strategy, that is, a strategy aimed at eliminating the aversive effect of the destabilization, rather than its causes. This is accomplished through an alternative commitment to a perceived stable meaning. A central point of this model is that the alternative meaning is non-specific – that is, it is not related to the destabilized meaning. What matters is that the new meaning restores a sense of stability to the individual's overall meaning system (hence the palliative nature of the strategy). In practice, the individual responds to destabilization like the person who, unable to finish the crossword puzzle, turns to watering the plants or putting the closet in order to regain a sense of being able to complete the task in which he or she engages. The authors point out that the model they developed allows them to integrate the diverse and divergent empirical findings in support of the various uncertainty theories. These findings can be interpreted as specific ways in which the palliative mechanism is expressed due to contextual conditions. As can be seen, the MMM does not merely note the empirical relationships between uncertainty and responses, nor does it account for that relationship because of the function they serve. Rather, it puts forward an argument about the intervening mechanism that leads the individual to respond in a certain way to uncertainty. Three aspects of this approach deserve to be highlighted:

(a) although obviously amenable to empirical verification, MMM conceptualization of the intervening mechanism is theory-driven – its elaboration is based on a strong theoretical framework – a theory of meaning, a psychological and neuroscientific model of the aversive neurophysiological activation, and of the conditions that supersede the palliative management of the aversive activation;

(b) the modeling of the intervening mechanism makes it possible to account for a particular feature of the response – its non-specificity. From this point of view, a reversal in the direction of reasoning can be recognized: it is not the feature of the response that determines the conjecture about the mechanism that produces it (see what was said previously about the a posteriori functionalist explanation adopted by most uncertainty theories); rather, it is the understanding of the intervening mechanism that makes it possible to understand the feature of non-specificity of the response;

(c) reference to a model of the intervening mechanism offers authors the opportunity to interpret a plurality of divergent empirical data in a unified way, integrating them into a more abstract and generalized explanation.

Considerations on the margin

Before concluding, we want to make two considerations prompted by the examples presented in the previous section.

First, modeling the intervening mechanism – the opening of the black box – requires a rethinking of the logic of explanation generally adopted as the foundation of scientific knowledge in the field of psychology. In most cases, the explanation of psychological phenomena is understood as the identification of links between causes and effects. The scientific experiment is, from this point of view, the methodological standard: ideally, by isolating the concurrence of other variables, it allows a causal relationship between independent and dependent variables to be established. Research often adopts articulated forms of this logic, involving reference to additional moderating and/or mediating variables; however, the underlying view of the standard of explanation as mapping causal relationships between variables remains valid.

This logic in psychology is widely used in spite of the conceptual criticisms of which it is a target. One cogent theoretical objection is that in the case of psychological phenomena concerning forms of subjectivity and the relationship between them and cultural contexts, variables do not describe separate and autonomous states endowed with the capacity to generate variations in energy-matter, in turn, capable of producing effects on other psychological variables (De Luca Picione & Salvatore, 2023). In short, psychological variables do not behave with each other like moving balls on the billiard table. On the contrary, the relationship between many psychological variables is semantic (Smedslund, 1988; for a discussion, see also Salvatore, 2020), grounded in cultural normativity (Harré & Gillett, 1994), and subservient to a part-whole logic (Valsiner, 2020). Variables are semantically related in the sense that, since they ultimately refer to processes of interpretation, the fact that psychological variable B follows variable A is to be understood in the sense that B is the interpretation – not the effect – of A (see in this regard what has been said about meaning as the sign that follows in Chapter 2). If Eleanor slaps John and the latter is offended and angry, the feeling of offense and anger is the way the slap is interpreted, not its effect – the effect of the slap is the flushed cheek. The normative basis of the relationship between the variables is a corollary of the semantic substance of that relationship – it is configured in terms of the cultural canons of the social group. This is the reason why Smedslund (1988) asserts that much research in psychology is *pseudoempirical*: it describes relationships between variables that are already an implicit part of the cultural norm at the foundation of common sense. Finally, again, as a corollary of the semantic nature of the relationship between psychological variables, they are expressions of part-whole relationships: they do not lend themselves to being considered separate entities in interaction with each other, but elements that participate in the same global dynamic of sensemaking (see in this regard the conceptualization of the meaning system as a network of signs, Chapter 2). From this point of view, when one considers variables as separate entities and then makes them interact, it is as if one considers the frame of a video a variable and treats the next frame as the effect of the previous one. Beyond the metaphor, consider the relationship between symbolic universes and other variables such as core values, sense of community, and description of one's cognitive style (Salvatore, Mannarini, et al., 2019). Such associations do not lend themselves to being interpreted as indicative of the fact that each symbolic universe influences other variables from the outside (or vice versa); rather, they should be seen as indicative of the fact that each symbolic universe is composed of a certain set of relationships between a set of signs – values, attitudes, cognitive styles, etc. – that can be represented at different levels of abstraction (on the representation of signs in terms of the level of abstraction, see Chapter 2, Section 5). There is no symbolic universe that causes adherence to a certain value system, a certain level of sense of community, a certain cognitive style, etc. – rather, the symbolic universe is the network woven by this set of signs.

The alternative to the search for discrete, cause-effect linkages is modeling, i.e., *the representation of the mode of functioning of the dynamic that fosters and shapes the evolution over time of phenomena in which it manifests itself*. In terms of the Aristotelian distinction, it is a matter of moving from the logic of efficient causality to the logic of formal causality, where the latter is the organization – the form – constituting the functioning of the object of investigation (for a discussion of the implications of this shift in psychology, see Heft, 2013). The referential activity theory offers an instructive example of such a logic – as noted previously, the description it proposes of the psychotherapeutic process does not call causal links into play. On the contrary, it describes an overall mode of functioning of the process, the latter understood as an organic totality unfolding over time – the cyclical alternation of phases of translation of one code into another – to which the interpretation of multiple phenomenal manifestations (e.g., therapist's interventions, their impact on the patient, quality of the alliance, etc.) is anchored.

Second, the referential activity theory, as well as the MMM model, show that the modeling approach to change implies the possibility of inscribing the understanding of the phenomena at stake in more general and abstract interpretive frameworks. The referential activity theory serves to conceptualize the therapeutic process. However, it is a more general model that returns an overall representation of the way the mind functions and the interaction between conscious and unconscious thought that underlies it. Similarly, the MMM view of the palliative response to aversive activation is used *locally* to understand the socio-cognitive response to uncertainty. However, it has a more general extension, encompassing the plurality of social settings and circumstances where the need to cope with aversive forms of neurophysiological activation is involved. This leads to the conclusion that there is no need to raise fences between the domains of intervention. On the contrary, it is legitimate to refer to a model of change that is just as abstract as object theory across domains of intervention. Such a model will, in turn, operate as a foundation for local theories that specify it within and by reason of specific field conditions that characterize single domains of intervention.

3 Is it worth opening the black box?

There are several reasons to believe that efforts to open the black box are worthwhile. One reason lies in the fact that the field of intervention does not always have, indeed quite rarely, clear and defined causal links such as that identified by Dr. Snow between the water dispenser and cholera contagion. Generally, the phenomena on which one intends to act have a field nature: they are a function of an interacting plurality of elements, which – taken singly – exert, at best, a limited impact on the phenomenon. To give a quantitative reference, consider that when in a research study, the explanatory variables explain a percentage of the variance of the dependent variable in the order of 25–30%; this is considered a satisfactory result.

Second, it should be borne in mind that the field nature of many psychological and psychosocial processes has, as a result, the fact that the ways the factors involved act on the phenomenon of interest may vary considerably from situation to situation (Salvatore & Valsiner, 2010). Consequently, factor-focused interventions encounter difficulties in being generalizable from one intervention situation to another.

Third, in the absence of an understanding of the mechanism of change, the intervention can only use – and therefore remain bound to – the ways in which the actors involved in it (clients, stakeholders) regulate the action affecting them. In other words, the psychologist operates within the *given context* (Grasso et al., 2016): their intervention utilizes – and therefore remains within – the system of semiotic resources already available within the field of intervention (see what was said previously about the pseudo empirical nature of much psychological research). As long as these resources are sufficient to fuel the intervention, this is not a problem; however, it becomes a problem in intervention contexts in which the available semiotic resources are insufficient to support the psychologist's action.

To clarify this central aspect, it may be useful to return to the book *Principles of Social Change* we referred to earlier (Jason, 2013). Based on direct and indirect experience accumulated over several decades of research and intervention, the North American author identifies five principles to which community development interventions should adhere: 1) determine the nature of the change being pursued so as to address the problem at the root; 2) identify the actors who have the power to influence the course of action related to the problem; 3) build coalitions with community actors who share the goals of the intervention; 4) exercise patience and perseverance, so as to value small progress, which is necessary to achieve long-term goals; and 5) verify results, so as to be clear about what has been done and what remains to be done. As a preliminary remark, we note that according to our proposed model of change (see Section 1), the five principles should be understood as *vectors*. From this perspective, Jason's book should more consistently be called: "Principles of Action to Promote Social Change." The central point we wish to highlight here, however, is another: *the effectiveness of these vectors is contingent on the presence of contextual resources that cannot be taken for granted.* Jason's proposed principles presuppose limiting ourselves to the elements that can be directly deduced from how they are formulated: a community context within which development goals enjoy a sufficiently broad level of consensus, a network of local powers that is neither overly fragmented nor overly rigid and hierarchical, and a civic infrastructure that allows for the support of the formation of alliances that are sufficiently stable to sustain medium-term goals.

All this leads to one conclusion: when the context of intervention already has the semiotic resources – social, institutional, organizational – necessary to nurture change, the intervention can also remain blind to the dynamic of change underlying the relational and social production of these resources. In many cases, however, such resources are not available, and therefore, the intervention cannot simply take the form of a sounded utilization of already given resources but rather must be configured as a device designed for their promotion. This requires an understanding of the psychosocial and cultural mechanisms generative of semiotic resources so that they can be activated and oriented in ways consistent with the objectives pursued. Intervention has to be thought of as *context to be constructed* rather than given.

4 Configurations of change. A typology

People's daily lives, social interactions, and institutions bear witness to the incessant evolution of meanings and how individual and social reality varies because of it. We accumulate information regarding facts and objects, we modify our opinions, and at certain times, we feel those close to us are the best in the world; at other times, we feel disappointed or angry with them; people quarrel for the most varied reasons and sometimes reconcile, they form couples, which sometimes last and sometimes do not; institutions introduce innovations, change organizational arrangements, and modify their policies. Variations can be point-like or incremental, unfolding in the space of minutes or decades, being recognizable or remaining beyond the threshold, being stable or unstable. Πάντα ρεῖ ὡσ ποταμόσ: the flow of meanings that shapes feeling, thinking, and acting is the living matter of individual and social worlds.

Two distinctions can help us map the proteiformity of life.

Forms of meaning

We can trace the content of sensemaking back to four general forms: *descriptions, judgments, procedures,* and *artifacts*. The distinction between descriptions and judgments reflects the conceptual analysis developed in the context of the philosophy of value (e.g., Zimmerman, 2015). By *description,* we mean a representation of a given object/event in terms of one or more attributes. "The Italian national soccer team won the 2021 European Championship" is a description that represents a state of affairs in terms of the relationship established between an object (the Italian national soccer team) and an attribute (being the winner of the 2021 European Championship). We group evaluative and deontic beliefs in *judgments*. An evaluative belief is a representation of the positive or negative value of the object to which it refers – for example, "Salerno is a beautiful city." A deontic-type belief is a representation of a canon that defines how things should be – for example, "human rights are inalienable." Values are a paradigmatic example of deontic belief (Hirose & Olson, 2015). It is worth adding that sometimes descriptions and judgments are intertwined so that the latter are conveyed by representations that have the shape of the former; this is the case when the description implies a value judgment – "Salerno is a city laden with art and history" – or where the description implies a violation of canon – "No-vaxers are a public health risk." *Artifacts* are meanings crystallized in the products of social action: objects (e.g., tools, art and design products, technology, forms of urban environment), devices (e.g., norms, organizational forms, commodities), and institutions (e.g., marriage, market, state, school). As activity theory has pointed out, all these products condense the meaning that governs and gives purpose to their production (Cole, 1996; see also Appadurai, 2013; Berger & Luckman, 1966). For example, a classroom with chairs placed in front of parallel rows of desks epitomizes the representation of the teacher-student relationship as one-way, one-to-many communication. Finally, by *procedures,* we denote the set of ways of operating and acting – procedural memories, ways of regulating emotions and thinking, and behavioral scripts. The choice to consider procedures as a semiotic element derives from the pragmatic and embodied conception underlying the theory of meaning adopted in this book (see Chapter 2). Controlling impulses, choosing clothes to wear, driving, going to a restaurant, and the implicit practices that regulate social exchange and life in organizations are all examples of this kind of procedural meaning, consisting of prereflexive habits that shape individual and collective behaviors.

It is worth pointing out that meaning change is not made experiential as such but always in terms of its impact on the forms of individual and social action: what we observe are the phenomenal markers of meanings, not the meanings. For example, we do not perceive that our neighbor has changed his way of representing us – what we perceive is that for some days now, he has been responding to our greeting in a more cordial way, engaging in conversation with us, seeking our gaze and showing appreciation for our jokes, etc.; from this, we infer that "internally" their image of us has changed: they now consider us worthy of greater interest and appreciation than until the recent past. Lastly, we relate to texts, combinations of signs of different kinds – bodily perceptions, words, sounds, images, bodily movements – from which we infer the meaning they express. This leads to the conclusion that texts are elements of phenomenal reality, while the four forms of meaning we have outlined previously are still within the latent domain of sensemaking – they are the arrows varying orientation shown in the grey part of Figure 3.1.

Forms and levels of abstraction of meaning. A typology

The four forms of meaning can be cross-referenced with the levels of abstraction discussed in Chapter 2 (Section 7), where we distinguished between *self-other affective schemes, hyper-generalizing signs, generalizing signs, collections,* and *singularities*.

Table 3.1 presents the typology obtained from the intersection. Cells report two types of meanings, one related to the field of individual experience – specifically, meanings related to neighborhood relationships (at the level of singularities and collections) and to a relationship with the community (at the level of generalized signs); the other related to the socio-institutional sphere – specifically, meanings related to activity as a university faculty (at the level of singularities and collections) and to a relationship with the institution (at the level of generalized signs). At the level of hyper-generalizing meanings, this distinction is lost; in fact, as we noted (Chapter 2, Section 6), at that level of abstraction, meanings are global, thus pertaining to the totality of the field of experience. At the even more abstract level of self-other schema, we find only procedural meanings, consistent with the fact that, at that level, meaning consists of patterns of bodily activation. Meanings reported in the grid are consistent with a positive connotation of the objects to which they refer; the

TABLE 3.1 Typology of semiotic elements

Level of abstraction	Descriptions	Forms of meaning		
		Judgments	Artifacts	Procedures
Singularity	"My neighbor is pleased to meet me."	"My neighbor is a courteous person."	Garage shared with neighbor	Subject greets neighbor amiably when they meet
	The university I work for has more than 800 years of history.	*The university I work for is prestigious.*	*The university logo*	*The lecturer spends most of the time in the office*
Collections	"My neighbors are satisfied with living in the neighborhood."	"My neighbors are polite people."	Condominium regulations	The neighborhood party is held every year to greet the arrival of spring
	Italian universities have been able to maintain levels of scientific productivity even in the face of significant reductions in public investment.	*The public university must be supported.*	*Ministerial investments to support young researchers*	*The use of colloquial language among faculty colleagues*
Generalized signs	"Crime rates are lower than average in the community."	"The community is a safe place."	Neighborhood associations	Civic engagement on the problems of the place where you live
	Institutions have made extensive use of flexible work arrangements to cope with the pandemic.	*I have trust in institutions.*	*The regulations linking the exercise of roles and professions to the possession of a degree*	*Adopt institutional rules to manage conflicts in the work context*
Hyper-generalized signs	"Acting according to justice is the most effective way."	"I have confidence in my surroundings."	The word agreement	Engage in human rights advocacy activities
Self-other affective schemes				Affectivization of reality as benign and nurturing

NB. In normal, the meanings are related to the individual and interpersonal sphere. In italics, the meanings are related to the socio-institutional sphere. Generalized meanings are underlined. In quotation marks, texts corresponding to declarative representations are expressible in terms of verbal statements. Unquoted texts refer to actions and devices.

table focuses on meanings of this type to highlight how the different levels of abstraction lend themselves to being considered progressive differentiations of an affective self-other schema: the affective state feeds representations that, as the level of abstraction is reduced, find anchorage in increasingly specific objects, yet retain their affective valence. This, among other things, implies that meanings of lower abstraction are nested within and thus also reproduce those of higher abstraction. For example, civic engagement in the community is a generalized sign of a performative nature (procedure) that simultaneously reflects a worldview (hyper-generalizing sign) and a form of affective semiosis (self-other schema).

Each of the meanings in Table 3.1 may go through a modification. For example, the person may come to the conclusion that the neighbor takes no pleasure in meeting them or that they are rude; the university logo may be redesigned; condominium rules changed, etc. Again, the person may feel their trust in institutions betrayed, as well as, even more generally, experiencing a reversal of the affective schema from benign and nurturing to a malignant and persecutory reality.

Modifications in meaning mapped by the typology are clearly not all of the same magnitude. The more generalized the meanings are, the more their modification invests in the identity and the sense of self. Since the subject (whether a person or social group) is defined in terms of the interpretation of the relationship it has with the world (see Chapter 2), the more extensive the modification of the interpretation of that relationship, the wider the domains of experience over which it unfolds, the more radical the change will be perceived to be. Changing the university's logo does not have the same identity value as plunging into a sense of generalized distrust of the world.

The extension of semiotic modification

Semiotic modifications deserve to be distinguished by reason of their extension. Reinforcing a belief by enriching it with arguments and data and changing it with the opposite belief are both forms of semiotic modification, however, of a different extension. This difference points back to the distinction that, with different concepts, a variety of authors have made between Level I and Level II change (e.g., Jason, 2013; Newman, 2000; Thompson & Hunt, 1996). In our view, however, it is appropriate to divide change into three levels rather than two, similar to what was proposed by Bateson, who, following his distinction between proto-learning (learning 1) and deutero-learning (learning 2), introduced the concept of learning 3, understood as a modification of the process of deutero-learning (Bateson, 1972). The latter is a learning that Bateson considers rare, related to special circumstances such as psychotherapy or peculiar religious experiences.

One patient, Mr. D., followed by one of us, spent a good part of his early sessions talking about his wife, how emotionally distant she had become from him, and how he considered this to be unfair, a betrayal that made him suffer and feel angry. In each session, the patient enriched his narrative of the affectively ungenerous wife with new details, including new episodes of marital and family life. Once, for example, he recounted how he felt humiliated and challenged by his wife, who at a dinner with friends a few days earlier had shown that she was enjoying herself, cheerfully participating in the conversation instead of thinking of him standing aside, unable to communicate with anyone. From that moment on, the belief about his wife was enriched with this additional provocative and derogatory valence, which was initially not present (level 1 learning). After a few months, the tenor of the accounts of the marital ménage went through a gradual modification – the patient had registered signs of a rapprochement with his wife, which made him feel less radically abandoned and alone, full of hope about the future of the relationship. Such a change is evidently of a different nature from the previous one. In this case, the representation of the wife varied in a more profound way than the type 1 learnings that had occurred up to that point – the belief modifies in sign, translating into an opposite version: the wife from evil stepmother is transformed into a prince charming. After a time to measured in years, the patient progressively broadened the point of view from which both beliefs recalled earlier – malignant wife and benign wife – were constructed and reproduced: the wife came to be interpreted, first cognitively, later also emotionally, not only and not mainly from the position of the one who expects to receive from the other, but also from the position of the one who gives to the other. From this new perspective, the patient began to perceive – to give value of life – and thus to explore his wife's problems: the debilitating impact of her violent recurring migraines, the work difficulties inherent in a profession characterized by a difficult interweaving of responsibility, precariousness, and dependence on political power, and the need to come to terms with their offspring's separation from the family unit. At this stage, the patient did not divest himself of the original point of view – namely, the focus on whether or not he was the object of the other's care, but he managed to alternate it with a new point of view – namely, representing the other as the object of care. This enabled him to gain more serenity toward himself and his wife, to rebuild within himself the desire toward his wife, to alleviate abandonment anxieties, and to increase his self-esteem; incidentally, all modifications had a positive impact on the marital ménage. This is level 3 of change: a shift in the point of view from which belief is constructed – in the terms used in Chapter 2: *a revision of the premises of meaning that configure the constitution of the object of experience.* Prior to this change, Mr. D. was moving within the one-dimensional semiotic field defined by the representation of the other as a source of care/love. The variability of that field was thus defined by the presence vs. absence of the other-who-loves. The other-as-object-of-care implies the emergence of a new dimension of the semiotic field: |giving vs. receiving care/love|. Because of this emergence, the previous variability of the patient's experience (benign vs. malignant wife) becomes an internal variability in one of the two polarities of the second dimension (the receiving polarity). The shift to the other polarity (giving) thus implies a relativization/reconfiguration of the original experience.

The triadic articulation of change illustrated previously can also be used at the meso- and macro-social levels. For example, the evolution of organizational models can be traced to make it indicative of the three levels of change. In the 1980s, organizations gradually adopted automated decision-making and management systems (CAD systems, *Computer Aided Design*), made possible by advances in information technology. The development of such systems took place in terms of the gradual increase in their ability to handle environmental variability through the incorporation of an increasing number of parameters and corresponding response alternatives. Such a development is an example of type 1 change: the CAD representation of environmental variability is progressively enriched with new parameters so as to expand the computational power of assimilating environmental inputs. However, this development found its limitation in the impossibility of expanding information processing capacity ad libitum. Above a certain threshold, the increase in the information load reduced the performance of processing systems rather than enhancing it (Pessa & Penna, 2000). A different approach emerged: lean production and demand orientation (Butera, 1991), which reversed the logical terms of the relationship between system and environment (type 2 change). CAD systems are an expression of the logic of *production orientation* – i.e., they take a predetermined repertoire of responses of the organization as a reference, defined on the basis of the internal architecture of the management and production system, and on that basis, they classify environmental inputs, so as to associate the latter with the former, according to the scheme: if (input), then (response). In contrast, lean production frees itself from the repertoire of predetermined responses to which it assimilates environmental variability and, in a sense, allows itself to be guided by the latter. It does this through the development of flexible organizational criteria and formats (e.g., reduction of hierarchical levels, network architecture) that enable the organization to prepare a rapid and effective response to environmental contingency (Mariotti, 1995). For example, the company does not define ex-ante the volumes and contents of production and then place products on the market but flexibly adapts production in response to fluctuations in demand. Roughly in the same years that the logic of customer orientation took hold, a further approach, termed *service orientation*, developed (Norman, 1986). The qualifying aspect of this model is the relational view of productive activity: service is a production process that uses the user as a factor of production. The user thus comes to be reinterpreted in terms of *prosumer*: producer and consumer at the same time. The logic of service has important conceptual and practical implications related to the weakening of organizational boundaries resulting from the co-opting of the customer in the production process. Here, we are interested in highlighting how service logic introduces a different type 3 change from the one related to the shift from production orientation to demand orientation. In fact, production orientation and demand orientation are internal variations on the same point of view: they share the dual view of production activity as an action composed of two separate and mutually independent entities, one of which assumes the function of regulating the other. The logic of service proposes a triadic view of production activity as a co-construction between provider and consumer, thus played out in the triangle formed by the two sub-jects and the context generated by their relationship (Ciavolino et al., 2017).

With reference to the macro-social plane, it is useful to recall the prevail-ing interpretation of populism (Kriesi & Pappas, 2015; see also Mannarini, Rochira, et al., 2020): a form of political platform that does not allow itself to be assimilated into the left-right dialectic historically underpinning political discourse. Populism is a "thin ideology" (Mudde, 2004), which is completed by assimilating, from time to time, due to the contexts and political actors that mobilize it, themes peculiar to the right (e.g., sovereignism) and/or the left (e.g., universal right to income). By reason of this definition, the evolu-tion of political thought internal to left and right discourses (e.g., the parti-tion of socialism between utopianism, Marxism, and social democracy) can be interpreted as a type 1 form of change, the cyclical evolution of consensus that alternately rewards right and left as a type 2 change, and the consensus garnered by populist discourse in certain historical phases, including the cur-rent one, as a type 3 change.

A structural model of semiotic change

Anticipating the computational approach that we will explore in more detail in the next chapter, in this section, we present a model of semiotic change that describes in dynamic-structural terms the qualitative distinction between type 1, 2, and 3 change proposed in the previous section. The model is based on the notion of the semiotic field introduced in Chapter 2. A semiotic field is a space whose structure is given by a number n of dimensions, each of which relates to a component of meaning. Figure 2.2 describes a semiotic field composed of two latent dimensions of meaning (the first two lines of semiotic force identi-fied by Salvatore and colleagues [2019b]: friend/foe, engagement/passivity). The relationship between these latent dimensions of sense and meanings – in this case, symbolic universes – are described geometrically in terms of their position in the semiotic field.

On this basis, we can conceptualize the three types of change in terms of the position of the interpreter in the semiotic field. This leads us to propose the distinction between *local variation, infrastructural change*, and *structural transformation*, corresponding to type 1, type 2, and type 3 change, respectively (for a similar view, see Grasso et al., 2016).

The sense-maker produces local variation in their own interpretive activity when the latter does not change its position within the semiotic field. This means that there is continuity in the premise of sense that shapes the interpretation of experience. The information and knowledge that this interpretation produces will, therefore, remain consistent and bound to the way the subject assimilates new environmental occurrences. For example, a person identified with the symbolic universe *ordered universe* who assumes as a premise of sense that what is right is also effective (see Chapter 2), will try to manage the conflict that has arisen with a colleague based on the assumption that it is always possible to find a solution that respects the motives of both and that this solution will also be the most effective. Again, in recent years, the populist narrative of the bad "élite" defending its own privileges against the good "people" has expanded, joining with the sovereigntist discourse that sees supranational institutions (primarily, the European Union) as an attack on national identity and autonomy. This is a local variation – the structure of meaning that substantiates populism has not changed: it has spread its reference to encompass even the techno-bureaucratic elite of supranational institutions. Further examples of this kind of movement constrained within the semiotic field are Mr. D. expanding his experience of his wife as aloof and malignant, the production paradigm fueling the development of CAD systems, and the internal evolution of left and right political thought. Ultimately, local variation in meaning is how the subject consolidates its interpretation, generating assimilative learnings of the new realities it experiences.

Instead, infrastructural modification implies a change in the position of the interpreter in the semiotic field. Salvatore and colleagues (2019b) discuss the symbolic universe of *others' world* – a worldview with which subjects are driven to identify themselves as a result of the failure of anchorage of sense provided by other symbolic universes – i.e., when the social reality undermines identification with interpersonal bond, with institutions, with the inherent rationality of things, and with the ingroup that other symbolic universes foster. That people can change symbolic universes over time is, moreover, indirectly evidenced by a datum: in a 2018 survey (Salvatore et al., 2018), the segment of the Greek population identified with the two symbolic universes expressing a fatalist and anomic worldview (*niche of belongingness* and *others' world*) proved to be 72%. It is hard to think of this figure as not reflecting the reaction of many Greeks to the deep social, economic, and institutional crises that have swept through that country for many long years. Mr. D. provides another example of infrastructural change as he begins to represent his wife as benign rather than malignant. Similarly, one can consider the shift from production to demand orientation, as well as the cyclical shift in consensus between left and right.

Structural transformation implies a change in the semiotic field: the subject's interpretive movement no longer stays within the premises given by the constitutive dimensions of the semiotic field but goes beyond the horizon of sense these dimensions offer and impose. In structural terms, this can be represented by the *change in the dimensions of the semiotic field*. It is in this sense that we speak of structural transformation – a change that goes beyond the structure given. On this, let's return to the semiotic field of symbolic universes illustrated in Chapter 2. Figure 2.2 depicts the semiotic field as two-dimensional. Actually, the analysis of the cultural milieu also identified a third dimension, interpreted by the authors as the form of demand: *demand for systemic resources* vs. *demand for identity/community* (see Chapter 2). To facilitate the exposition, we have not previously mentioned this. Now, in contrast to the other three symbolic universes, *ordered universe* and *caring society* are also associated with such a third dimension of meaning: the *ordered universe* is substantiated by the combination of friendship/engagement/demand for identity/community; *caring society* by the combination of friendship/engagement/demand for systemic resource. Thus, a person who was to change their identification from one of the three two-dimensional symbolic universes to one of the two three-dimensional symbolic universes would achieve a structural transformation. When Mr. D. goes beyond seeing himself as the target of the desire of the other person, he adds a dimension of meaning to his own semiotic field: being the source of the desire of the other person. The same argument can be made in the case of service orientation, which introduces into the semiotic field of management theory and practice the dimension of producer-user co-construction. Again, populism adds the elite vs. people dimension to the unidimensional semiotic field of political thought, traditionally based on left-right opposition.

5 The mechanics of change

Background

This section focuses on the mechanism of change. The following discussion develops from a general theoretical assumption that it is appropriate to make explicit: *semiotic change is not a process separate from the more general dynamic of sensemaking*. On the contrary, semiotic change is the way in which the dynamic of sensemaking unfolds. Consequently, semiotic change must be understood on the basis and in terms of the general model of the dynamic of sensemaking.

A paradigmatic example of this logic is the Piagetian theory of cognitive development. This theory explains the process of progressive construction of different mental structures during ontogeny as the emergent product of a single fundamental dynamic – the balance (equilibration) between assimilation and accommodation. Another example of such an approach is provided by the theory of referential activity to which we have already referred – it explains the therapeutic process in terms of a general model of the mind (the multiple code theory). These examples illustrate how *change is a variation fostered by the invariant mode of functioning of the fundamental dynamic*. Consistently, the following discussion will consider semiotic change as the form that the dynamic of sensemaking takes under certain conditions (catalyzers). In other words, the dynamic of sensemaking does not change; it always operates in the same way, according to the same rule (invariance), and, for that very reason, takes different forms.

This is a general principle of a theoretical-methodological order, which we might call *bifocality*: every variation is the form by which an invariance of a higher logical order is reproduced. Consequently, understanding change requires both recognizing what varies and the more general process that is reproduced through that variation. For example, saying "1, 2, 3, 4" is an exercise of variation (the digits are different). At the same time, such variation is the way the action of counting is reproduced. The principle of bifocality harks back to Maturana and Varela's (1980) distinction between structure and organization: organization is the way the parts of the system relate to each other to reproduce the structure – when perturbed, the system causes the organization to vary in order to preserve the structure.

At the heart of the dynamic

What drives people, social groups, and institutions to vary their interpretive activity in order to preserve the underlying system of meaning?

The embodied, pragmatist view of cognition developed in the last quarter century (e.g., Barsalou, 1999, 2008; Gallagher, 2005; Engel et al., 2015) supplies the tools to formulate an answer to this question. According to this view, cognitive processes serve action. It follows that in order to model cognitive processes, it is necessary to understand what demands the regulation of action places on cognition.

Authors who have moved in this direction have conceptualized cognition as the process of constant modulation of the instantaneous state of the body by which the organism represents to itself, in real-time, the variations in interaction with the environment. The basic operating principle of cognition – if you like, its ultimate goal – is to maintain that interaction in the equilibrium condition necessary to act in and through the environment. In short, cognition consists of the production of sensorimotor maps of the moment-by-moment variations in the states of the environment to maintain action coupled with the environment.

A central aspect implied in such a view is that *mapping of environmental variations must necessarily be anticipatory*: action regulated on knowledge of what has already happened would imply too long a time frame, incompatible with the demands of fine regulation of the coupling, therefore of adaptation, and more generally of survival. The gazelle cannot wait for the lion to start chasing it to start running.

Cognition thus behaves like a meteorologist rather than a notary – it forecasts the coming environmental state rather than taking note of what has happened. More precisely, it is a Bayesian type of prediction (Barsalou, 2011), i.e., an inference guided by a priori knowledge about the range of possible developments of the environment. Consider a tennis player: if his movements were triggered at the point where it is appropriate to hit the ball, the racket would reach that point when the ball was already beyond it. Fortunately for the tennis player, his movement starts earlier, thanks to the prediction of where the ball will be a few tenths of a second later. Even without having played tennis, every one of us has experienced the anticipatory nature of mental activity: it will have happened to all of us to involuntarily collide with an object when it has come to an unexpected halt or slowed down. Such kinds of events show how the adjustment of the trajectory and speed of our movement is calculated not as a function of the actual position of the object but based on the anticipation of its position at the next moment. Unintended collision is the consequence of the failure of such anticipation. Feints in football are another example of the anticipatory nature of prediction: with the feint, the attacker provides the defender with an environmental input that triggers in the defender an erroneous prediction of the attacker's trajectory. The defender will thus be induced to move in a direction that will favor, rather than hinder, the attacker's movement. Not surprisingly, every good defender knows that in order not to fall into the trap of feints, one must look at the ball and not at the attacker's body.

Thus, the cognitive system – broadly understood as a mind/body unit – is constantly searching for successful prediction – hereafter: *fit*. The search for fit is an asymptotic effort – the continuous variation in the environment means that every prediction needs to be constantly updated so as to preserve fit. Moment by moment, the cognitive system compares the prediction produced in the previous moment and the current input to which it refers. In the case of deviation (*misfit*), the sensorimotor pattern is reshaped to recover the fit. The greater the *misfit* between prediction and current input, the greater the amount of sensorimotor activation required to recover the fit. Consider a person lying on the lawn and engaged, like Herman Hesse's Peter Camenzind, in contemplation of the shapes assumed by the clouds in the sky. At some point, an object – a bumblebee – enters Peter's field of vision. Up to that point, grappling with the minimal changes in the field of vision induced by the slow movement of the clouds, the search for the fit had required Peter to do minimal work to adjust. Peter could use contemplation to relax. The appearance of the bumblebee introduces a local fall in fit, which forces Peter to do additional cognitive work necessary to recover the fit – moving his head, refocusing his gaze, recruiting mnestic traces useful for recognition, etc.

In the search for fit, the cognitive system moves following a principle of economy – the search is carried out through the sensorimotor response that requires the least expenditure of energy (for a discussion of the neurobiological basis of this principle, see Friston, 2010). This results in a hierarchy of changes in the responses used to maintain coupling with the environment, which can correspond to the three types of change discussed previously.

1. In the case where the trajectory of environmental states is maintained within a narrow margin of variability, that is, within the space of variation mapped by the a priori knowledge underlying Bayesian inference, the fit is maintained through fine modulations of sensorimotor responses. The resulting stability allows the establishment of associative links between individual responses and thus the consolidation of learning to which we referred previously with the term *local variation*. Consider, for example, a tennis player who, in training, repeatedly receives the ball the same way again and again to stabilize by repetition the sequence of instantaneous micromovements that make up the stroke to be perfected.

2. In other cases, environmental variability exceeds the margin defined by a priori knowledge. In that situation, prediction based on the a priori knowledge of the possible evolution of the environment fails. This results in the variation being a *global variation*: what changes is not a contingent state of the given environment but the environment as a whole. Consequently, *misfit* recovery must be accomplished by the modification of the a priori knowledge rather than, as in the previous case, the use of that knowledge. This evidently requires higher energy expenditure since interaction with a global variation in the environment involves calling up equally global sensorimotor responses. For example, take a person who meets an acquaintance and strikes up a conversation. Up to a certain point, the discussion proceeds in a friendly manner within the space of variation mapped by the person's a priori knowledge of that type of environment. The sensorimotor mapping of the interaction proceeds in a regime of stability of the capability of anticipations to retain fit. At some point, the acquaintance pulls a gun out of their jacket and points it at the other person – such an event is not anticipated by the a priori knowledge of the relational environment. To recover the fit, the person who has become the target will not be able to simply produce modulations of their own sensorimotor response: they will

have to redefine the context of the interaction, from friend to enemy. They will have to make a change to the values of the defining parameters of the a priori knowledge on which the Bayesian prediction about what is happening is based. This is the level of response variation corresponding to the *infrastructural change*.

3. There are reasons to agree with Bateson's proposal to introduce an additional level of variation. This occurs when, according to the terminology adopted here, changing the value of the a priori knowledge is not sufficient for effective predictions to be made. In such cases, a priori knowledge will have to be redefined structurally, i.e., by changing the type of parameters that define it rather than the parameter values. Changing the type of parameters corresponds to what we called *structural change* in the previous section – it corresponds to making other dimensions of the variability of the environment relevant rather than those previously used. Therein lies the difference with the type of variation in the previous point: the variation consisting of changing the values of the parameters of the a priori knowledge is kept within the given environmental variability. For example, the evolution of a friendly environment may range from remaining friendly to turning unfriendly. The variation of the type of parameters results in a higher-order logical change: the emergent environment comes to be configured because of additional dimensions of variability, those introduced by the new parameters of the a priori knowledge. Incidentally, the variation of the type of parameters can either increase or decrease. The examples we presented in the previous section indicate structural transformations realized through an increase in the dimensionality of the representation; in other cases, however, the transformation is realized in the opposite way, through a reduction in dimensionality.

Semiotic change is the way of stabilizing the premises of sense

The embodied idea of cognition as a search for fit can be connected to the triadic theory of sensemaking. As we have already pointed out (see Chapter 2, Section 2), semiosis is embodied: signs are ultimately conceptualizable as sensorimotor patterns. Even signs of an abstract nature are conceivable in this way: as material elements associated in a sufficiently established way with a class of sensorimotor responses (what specific response will be activated among them depends on the context) (Borghi et al., 2017). Take the following word as an example:

DOG

What we perceive is a distribution of color on the sheet. This perception consists of a pattern of sensorimotor activation that is, in turn, associated with a class of further responses (e.g., the response that substantiates the annoying thought of having to take the dog for his afternoon walk). As evidenced by Embodied Cognition, this class of responses shares many somatic processes with that elicited by direct perception of a dog. From this perspective, the DOG sign is a surrogate for such perception (Clark, 2005), a way of replacing the percept with another material element that elicits an equivalent sensorimotor response (recall in this regard the Peircean notion of the correspondence relation between signs, see Chapter 2, Section 1). Thanks to surrogates, the subject acquires the freedom to generate the world of experience semiotically – that is, they need not encounter one of those four-legged barking and sometimes biting animals in the flesh to have (a surrogate) experience of them; it is enough for the subject to mobilize the surrogate sign. Therein lies the fundamental evolutionary advantage that humans have achieved with the emergence of language – acquiring autonomy over environmental contingencies through the mediation of a system of signs that can be manipulated recursively (Corballis, 2011), i.e., that can be mobilized at will, to order them into infinite trajectories, each constituting a surrogate environment. Ultimately, such manipulation de-anchors the organism from the instantaneous state of the environment (Valsiner, 2007): the organism does not respond to the immediate environmental input but to its interpretation, i.e., to the surrogate signs that it is capable of mobilizing.

The previous example gives conceptual substance to the parallelism between the Peircean model of affective semiosis and that of sensorimotor response remodulation. Response remodulation aimed at prediction fit preservation corresponds, in the language of triadic sign theory, to the stabilization of the ground operated through the activation of equivalent signs that reproduce over time the correspondence between the representamen and the dynamic object. In short, the conservation of fit is the sensorimotor correlate of the semiotic value of the sign (see Chapter 2, Section 6): the reproduction over time of the ground. If you will, the conservation of fit is the engine that fuels the incessant dynamic of stabilizing the premises of sense at the foundation of the social action.

This leads us to the following conclusion: *semiotic change is a function of the regulation of the social action*. The dynamic of sensemaking fosters trajectories of signs whose fit reflects the subject's need to retain the stability of the premises of sense that make the sequence determined up to that moment interpretable. In the final analysis, the fit consists of this condition of interpretability of signs and, thus, of coordination of action.

The three structural levels of semiotic change thus reflect the degree of change in the trajectory of signs necessary to preserve the stability of the premises of sense/ground. If social action is maintained within – and thus fosters the stability of – the premises of sense, the chain of signs does not need to introduce changes in the equivalence nexuses placed at its foundation. This means that both the defining quality of the ground and the specific state/degree of that quality (henceforth, for brevity: state) remain constant and, as such, work as the foundation of the coordination of the action. Consequently, the action will consist of a sequence of signs, each of which associates an additional element with the state of the quality, thus enriching the information associated with it. As should be clear from the preceding discussion, this is the level of semiotic change to which we have referred with the term *local variation*. For example, consider the following sequence of signs: |my car|; |is hybrid-powered|; |has low fuel consumption|, |high performance|, |easy to drive|. The ground that this sequence reproduces is the quality consisting of being a device with structural and functional attributes. Furthermore, what characterizes the ground is that positive states are attributed to this quality. A possible further sign that can be added to such a sequence, without thereby altering the ground, could be: |has resistant mechanics|. This further association results in the learning of additional information. Such learning does not alter the ground; on the contrary, it occurs precisely because of the stability of the latter.

In cases where an incoming sign does not lend itself to be interpreted in the light of the given premises of sense (return to the gun suddenly extracted and pointed at the interlocutor during the friendly discussion), this destabilizes the premises. The next sign will therefore have to remodel the ground to restore the fit. The remodulation of the ground will follow the principle of economy recalled in the previous paragraph: it will operate primarily in terms of varying the state of quality, leaving the quality unchanged. Indeed, such a variation requires less cognitive work since it moves within the interpretive context defined by the quality at that important moment. The dynamic of sensemaking thus enters the condition of *infrastructural modification*. For example, consider that one adds |it nevertheless has an inefficient electronic apparatus|, |bad roadholding|, or |poor bodywork| to the sequence of signs given previously in relation to the car. In this case, the premise of sense (the ground) could not remain on the positivity of the car's structural and functional attributes, but it will have to shift to its opposite or at least maintain itself on an intermediate position between positive and negative. In this case, therefore, there would be a remodulation of the ground, however, leaving as given the relevant quality ("functional device") as a variation from one to another of the states that this quality can assume. It should be added, and this is an important point, that the quality whose states are varied can be represented on one of several levels of abstraction discussed in Chapter 2 and recalled previously (see Table 3.1) – the more abstract and generalized the level at which the rewriting of the premise maps, the greater its polarized nature. In the example referring to the car, the rewriting of the ground is carried out on the level of singularity or collection (depending on whether we are talking about a specific car or referring to the category of cars to which the specimen belongs). Given the limited level of generalization, such grounding lends itself to continuous modulation – it does not necessarily present itself in terms of the juxtaposition of positive and negative; on the contrary, it also admits intermediate positions. As we noted previously, when the first signs that refer to positive attributes of the device are succeeded by signs that recall negative attributes, the quality "functional device" need not imply a radical inversion of attribute – it could remain in an intermediate zone, which makes possible further signs of both positive and negative valence. It is a different matter when the ground is defined at the level of more abstract signs (generalized, hyper-generalized signs, and affective self-other schemes) – in these cases, the variation in the ground takes on progressively more polarized forms. Consider the example of the acquaintance who draws his gun – here, the variation is from a friendly state to its opposite. From this point of view, the polarities of the semiotic lines of force presented in Chapter 2 can each be seen as a dimension of bimodal variability of a ground consisting of generalized and polarized affective valence – e.g., from a friendly world to an enemy world.

Humor lends itself to exemplifying the shift from one polarity to the other. Consider the following joke:

Wife: "Dear, today is our anniversary. We've been married 25 years. Have you thought about how to celebrate?"
Husband: "I thought of taking you to the United States."
Wife: "Wow! . . . And what will you do when we get to 50 years?"
Husband: "I'll come and pick you up."

Until the moment before the husband's last statement, the sequence of signs activates and reproduces a ground consisting of the marital relationship and its attribute of positivity. The final sentence reverses that attribute by 180°, and with that inversion forces a reversal of the meaning of the entire previous sequence – the husband intends to push his wife away, not to build with her a moment of sharing; the 25 years of union is not a positive event to be celebrated but a time that must be prevented from lingering; the wife's enthusiasm is not a sign of the value of the relationship but of her inability to perceive the state of the relationship. The affective activation with which the pleasure of the joke is substantiated is the cue of the sensorimotor response that retroactively reconstructs the stability of the sense premise.

Finally, in the context of what has been discussed so far, *structural transformation* corresponds to the radical rewriting of the ground – it is not only the state of the quality that varies, but the quality itself. Returning to the considerations presented in Chapter 2 about the role played by the ground in the constitution of experience, modifying the quality operating as ground involves redefining the field of experience – it is not the values attributed to the object that vary, but the object itself. The considerations about the different levels of abstraction on which the modification of ground can take place also apply here. Let us return to the sequence of signs relating to the car. Imagine that it continues with a sign such as: |it's beautiful| (or with its opposite |it's ugly|) or |it's a present I gave myself for my fiftieth birthday|, or again: |these Germans! how they make cars . . . |. All these signs are outside the ground "functional device," they cannot be interpreted by means of a variation of its attributes. Their interpretation requires a rewriting of the ground, with the pertinentization of a different quality – the aesthetic appearance, being the object of one's desire, or the Germans' skills. As already mentioned, these grounds are placed on a low level of abstraction, so their variation does not affect the whole of the relationship between the subject and the world. The case is different when what varies is the ground defined by signs placed on a higher level of abstraction. Moving from the left-right axis to that of populism is a change that reshapes the premise of sense that profoundly constitutes politics: for those who assume such a ground, where before there were institutional actors engaged in designing and implementing policies, now there is an elite opposed to the people. Similarly, changing from identification with the symbolic universe *interpersonal bond* to that of *caring society* does not consist solely and primarily in a change at the level of content – indeed, both such universes have a positive worldview – as much to a change in the object of experience one relates to: in one case what one "sees" are interpersonal ties and their emotional vicissitudes, in the other institutional transactions among social actors.

To illustrate this last point, consider the following situation:

> A pedestrian is crossing the street on the crosswalk. The car stops and gives them the right of way. The pedestrian thanks them with a wave of the hand and a smile.

It could be said that the pedestrian thanks them because they are polite and, with this gesture, they express their appreciation and gratitude to the motorist. All this may be true, but it is not sufficient to understand what happened. The pedestrian's good manners help us to explain that the pedestrian feels obliged to express their gratitude/appreciation. Yet, such feelings are made possible by the fact that the pedestrian's experience of crossing is that of being a person in relation to another person, with the latter showing courtesy. In other words, the grateful pedestrian experiences an interpersonal relationship and interprets it with the affective (gratitude/appreciation) and pragmatic (thanking) meanings typical of that field of experience. However, such an experience is not a record of a fact. Rather, it reflects the constitution of a dyadic ground – the interaction between the two people – as the object of the experience. For example, a different ground would be possible: the pedestrian considers themselves and the driver in relation not with each other but both with the institutional system that regulates road traffic. The experience constituted by this triadic ground would not be of two interacting individuals (quality) performing a ritual of interpersonal courtesy (the state of the quality) but of institutional actors both in relation to a general norm. Within such a premise of sense, the mobilization of semiotic resources peculiar to dyadic social contexts – good manners, feelings of gratitude – would prove to be clearly inappropriate.

Summary

Given the complexity and articulation of the discussion put forward in this section, a summary of its main points may be useful.

Our arguments can be broken down into the following points.

1. Semiotic change is the way in which the dynamic of sensemaking operates. This means that the dynamic of sensemaking does not change. What does change is the trajectory of signs through which that dynamic is reproduced over time.

2. What drives the dynamic of sensemaking to change the trajectory of signs (which sign comes after which sign), making up change, is the need to keep the premise of sense at the foundation of the interpretation of signs stable, and with it the possibility of regulating the action.

3. On the micro-processual level, the stability of the premise of sense lends itself to be conceptualized in terms of preserving the fit of the Bayesian anticipatory interpretation of environment variation. In terms of the semiotic theory, the stability of that premise consists of the reproduction over time of the ground through the mobilization of signs that preserve the relation of correspondence between the original representamen and the dynamic object.

4. Variation in the trajectory of signs can take many forms, which we have traced back to the three structural levels – *local variation, infrastructural change,* and *structural transformation*. It can also be mapped at different levels of abstraction; the greater the level of abstraction involved, the more polarized the change involved.

5. The kind of change that takes place depends on the extent of the destabilization of the premises of sense/ground. In this regard, we have distinguished between the ground that remains stable, the ground destabilized at the level of the degree/state of its quality, and the ground destabilized at the level of its quality. We have thus put these three forms of destabilization in correspondence with the three structural levels of change – local variation, infrastructural change, and structural transformation, respectively.

6. This correspondence is due to the fact that the rewriting of the ground follows an optimization principle – the subject tries to maintain as much of the

given balance as possible, mobilizing cognitive work to rewrite only what is necessary.

Ultimately, semiotic change is the way the dynamic of sensemaking both adapts and fosters action. To produce semiotic change, the action must be modified, that is: the field of interaction between actors to which the dynamic of sensemaking is commensal must be modified.

Before concluding, two observations are useful.

1. The three levels of change can be connected to the distinction between *significance in praesentia* and *in absentia* (see Chapter 2). Local variation and infrastructural change are forms of within-ground variation concerning the significance *in praesentia*: the establishment of associative links between signs that can be represented. Structural transformation, on the other hand, is a form of between-ground variation; as such, it refers to the significance *in absentia*. As we will have a chance to discuss later, psychological intervention extends its interest in all three types of change but defines its specificity at the level of the *significance in absentia* – several other forms of professional intervention (e.g., teaching) share, with psychology, action at the level of local variation and infrastructural change; psychology has distinctive models of analysis and action related to structural transformations.
2. The model of semiotic change we have presented is ultimately based on the view of the dynamic of sensemaking as an operationally closed system (Maturana & Varela, 1980). Sensemaking adapts itself constantly to preserve the stability of its foundations. It does not change exogenously as a consequence of the environmental stimulus in that it does not learn from what is external to it. Rather, it rewrites the premise of sense on which it operates so as to reproduce itself: it modifies the organization (semiotic change) to preserve its structure (fit capacity). It follows that semiotic change cannot be exported. What psychological intervention can do is create conditions of action such that premises of sense are destabilized, and thus, subjects are induced to rewrite them. Psychological intervention, to put it in the terminology of autopoietic systems theory (Maturana & Varela, 1980), is perturbative, not instructive.

6 Catalyzers of change

As shown by the discussion developed in the previous section, semiotic change is the way in which the dynamic of sensemaking reorganizes in the face of the continuous perturbation induced by the moment-by-moment change in the interaction with the environment. This general conclusion raises a relevant question: if, as discussed previously, change can vary in extension (local variation, infrastructural mutation, structural transformation), what aspect of perturbation determines that difference?

In the previous section, we gave an initial answer to this question, arguing that the destabilization induced by the perturbation can have different timing and that, due to this difference, the dynamic of sensemaking either does not vary the ground/premise of sense (local variation), or varies the degree/state of quality (infrastructural change), or varies the quality (structural transformation). However, this response needs to be further articulated to specify the characteristics of the environment that substantiate the variable extent to which it perturbs the dynamic of sensemaking. This is what we aim to do in this section.

The tendency to simplify through abstraction

First, a structural feature of the dynamic of sensemaking should be recalled: its self-referential nature. As repeatedly discussed in this and the previous chapter, the dynamic of sensemaking operates as an operationally closed system – that is: *its purpose is to reproduce itself, not to generate knowledge about the environment.* The informational power of the dynamic of sensemaking is a by-product, so to speak, a kind of side effect generated by the incessant activity of stabilizing itself in which that dynamic is engaged. As we have already noted (Section 5), the metric of the effectiveness of this stabilization is the amount of energy mobilized by the subject to keep fit: *the dynamic of sensemaking responds to perturbation with the minimum amount of semiotic change that is necessary for the purposes of maintaining stability.*

The manifestations of the tendency to respond to the destabilization of meaning in a conservative way, in terms of simplifying the variability of the environment rather than making it more complex, are innumerable. It will have happened to all of us to do as Michelangelo did with his Moses and more or less metaphorically hurl the hammer at the object whose performance did not yield to our intentions. How many times have we perceived rejection as an offense/attack perpetrated against us, even when expressed politely and amply justified? Proverbs such as "don't throw the baby out with the bathwater" and "you can't judge a book by its cover" are ways to warn about the risks of simplified interpretations of social relations. Simplification does not only affect people: the contemporary political and institutional sphere is traversed by oversimplified forms of thought and discourse – for example, conspiracy, fake news, homogenization of scientific knowledge to opinions, and blindness to climate change. In the words of Umberto Eco,

> Social media give speech rights to legions of imbeciles who used to speak only at the bar after a glass of wine, without harming the community. They

were immediately silenced, while now they have the same right to speak as a Nobel Prize winner. It is the invasion of imbeciles.

(https://www.lastampa.it/cultura/2015/06/11/
news/umberto-eco-con-i-social-parola-
a-legioni-di-imbecilli-1.35250428/)

The recent film *Don't Look Up* is a powerful illustration of the preference for stabilizing simplified beliefs rather than enhancing their informational capacity. Two American scientists discover that an asteroid will soon impact Earth, resulting in the extinction of human life on the planet. Invited to tell a widely watched television program about the discovery, they are expected to simplify the news, stripping it of all technicalities so as to treat it as a topic of conversation, somewhere between gossip and the sentimental drama of a musical duo. The very title of the film is emblematic: "don't look up" is the slogan of the President's political platform, which proposes priorities other than the need to save humankind from extinction – if you avoid seeing the asteroid, it's not there; the opposite of the well-known anti-AIDS campaign slogan of a few years ago.

The literature on socio-cognitive response to uncertainty offers much data consistent with what happens in everyday life – as we have already noted (Chapter 2), when exposed to uncertainty, people tend to embrace simplified beliefs based on ingroup-outgroup polarization. Moreover, as pointed out by the *Maintenance Meaning Model* (Proulx & Inzlicht, 2012), the response is palliative: it serves to restore the stability of the meaning system, not to actually resolve the criticality that the destabilized meaning has encountered. In the terms used previously, the dynamic of sensemaking is primarily concerned with restoring its own stability, not with enhancing its informational capacity through accommodation to the destabilizing environmental input.

Without claiming to be exhaustive, we can observe that many forms of simplification present a fundamental characteristic: they absolutize one component of the object to which the belief refers, "devitalizing" the others, that is, the informational components associated with the aspects backgrounded. This operation of abstraction is accomplished by subjugating the belief to the class of meaning that fosters the salience of the absolutized component. When I pick on the poor fountain pen that is not doing its duty, angrily slamming it against the table as if to punish it, this happens because what I experience of the pen is exclusively its being an object that frustrates my desire. Its functional components of social and economic value and so forth, do not fall within my field of experience and, therefore, do not impact my actions. As a result, I am not in a position to perceive the possibility of acting on the pen to recover its functionality or to avoid the damage that I do to it – and, therefore, to me, its owner – by my Michelangelesque gesture. As in the example just given, sometimes the generalized class of meaning made salient is affect-laden; at other times, it is a social norm (itself rooted in the affective sense of one's own identity belonging). On this, think of the classic studies on conformism that show that people prefer to follow the President's suggestion not to look up, lest they learn a piece of information that would undermine their sense of group belonging. The reign of fake news in public communication can be understood in this sense: people do not mobilize signs to produce and use knowledge but to generate discursive rituals capable of fostering the sense of belonging of the participants in that ritual. People identify with the common belief; the more that belief is detached from the facts of reality, the more it is able to differentiate believers and non-believers, thus operating as an identity marker. Believing that the earth is flat, that vaccines are a manipulation by governments, that aliens have taken over world institutions, and that Juventus has stolen all the championships it has won are semiotic passports that give access to one of the many tribes that recognize themselves by virtue of their taking root in a territory of the imaginary. Even the field of science is not immune to simplifying abstraction. Reportedly, Einstein rejected quantum theory on the grounds that the latter violated the ordered conception of the universe at the basis of physics at the time – God does not play dice. As Kuhn (1970) helped us to understand, scientific paradigms define the boundary of the thinkable and plausible through the backgrounding of data radically at odds with normal science (e.g., the nonlocal causality form of quantum correlation). In books by Chinese astronomers working in the period corresponding to our own Middle Ages, comets are described that their contemporary European astronomers did not record – this evidently was not because of an epidemic of blindness but rather as a result of the fact that the European Ptolemaic view was not compatible with the perception of a luminous body moving across the celestial vault. *Don't Look Up* is not just a sign of our times.

Incidentally, it is worth pointing out that the tendency to simplify is not necessarily an alternative to complication. On the contrary, many simplifying theories are complicated. Consider, for example, how articulate conspiracy theories can be and how many intermediate conjectures they resort to as the semiotic silicone needed to hold the pieces of belief together. Even theories produced in normal science contexts tend progressively to become more complicated with the addition of ad hoc hypotheses that operate as a protective buffer aimed at neutralizing the destabilizing impact of conflicting data (Lakatos, 1978). The complication of simplification is thus not an oxymoron: as the concept is used here – in structural terms – the opposite of simplification is not complication, but complexity – that is, the multidimensionality of aspects that the map of the object takes into account.

Simplification and social bonding. The Pentecost effect

The logical error of judging the tendency of the dynamic of sensemaking to produce simplified forms of meaning as dysfunctional is due to the undesirability of their outcome. The undesirability of phenomena such as conspiracy theories, fake news, and the aggressive response to the experience of the limiting of desire – in the very many forms that such a response takes, from quarreling over parking to genocide – concerns the social and ethical plane. The process of semiotic change is not related to that plane – it is an intrinsic quality of the organization of life, no different from the force of gravity. Just as we do not consider the latter negative because, in some cases, people fall out of windows and planes crash; similarly, semiotic change should not be considered critical because, in some cases, it produces socially undesirable outcomes. On the other hand, beyond its socially problematic manifestations, the tendency of the dynamic of sensemaking to simplify underlies the very possibility of social bonding. As we have repeatedly pointed out (see Chapter 2), action is based on shared premises of sense. It is the sharing of such premises that makes it possible for actors to reduce the margins of mutual variability and thus coordinate action (Salvatore et al., 2006/2009). Carli (1987a, 1987b) called such sharing *collusion*, particularly in its affective component, highlighting its foundational function of the social bond.

Now, as noted, the generalized signs that substantiate the premises of sense are significances *in absentia*: they operate as the foundation of the social bond precisely because they are not the object but the condition of the interpretation. Thus, the sharing of premises of sense among actors cannot take place through negotiation. Collusion is not the outcome of a stipulation. Nor can it be the outcome of habit since the latter results from the repetition of a given course of action, which in turn must be based on shared premises of sense, in a *regressus in infinutum*: to share premises needs action, for there to be action, shared premises are needed, and so on. The self-referentiality of the dynamic of sensemaking resolves this logical paradox. Actors do not share the premise of sense in that they do not adhere to the same meaning; rather, each actor adheres to their own premise of sense, which – precisely because of sensemaking's tendency to simplify – is compatible with that of the other actors. Actors, therefore, do not share but rather *compatibilize* (we apologize for the term but could not find a better one) each other's own premise of sense. We propose a model of how this happens in what follows (for a discussion, see Salvatore, 2016c; see also Cremaschi et al., 2021; Salvatore, De Luca Picione et al., 2022).

First, it should be noted that each actor dances alone: each follows the music of their own music sheet. They do so even if they believe they are dancing in pairs or groups. Subjectivity is inherently monadic. This consideration follows directly from the self-referential nature of sensemaking. Each actor is able to assimilate any environmental input into the generalized system of meanings with which they identify. This is due to the oppositional structure of generalized signs (i.e., domain beliefs, worldviews, self-other affective schemas). Because of this structure, the subject can always use signs to interpret experience, as any environmental input will be associated with one polarity or the opposite: it's six of one and half a dozen of the other. For example, if the subject is identified with the affective dimension of evaluating the environment's ability to generate pleasure, then any environmental occurrence will be signified as pleasant (if the occurrence is associated with body states of that type) or, if not, as unpleasant. Incidentally, such a bimodal mechanism of affective semiosis underlies Melanie Klein's conceptualization of the infant's subjective experience in the early stages of life, characterized by the schizo-paranoid position. The infant symbolizes the present mother as a good object; her absence is not perceived as such, but as the presence of the bad object, i.e., the absence is not represented as a negation of the mother's presence (mother is not present), but as an activation of the opposite affective polarity: the presence of the bad mother. More generally, the oppositional structure of generalized signs and the role it plays in assimilating experience is a computational model that corresponds to the psychoanalytic idea that the unconscious does not consider negation (Freud, 1900/1953; Matte Blanco, 1975).

But then, if everyone dances alone, each locked in their own self-referentiality, how is the coordination of social action possible? Our answer is, only in a seemingly paradoxical way, coordination emerges precisely because of self-referentiality. To understand this, what has already been noted in Chapter 2 must be considered: the affective self-other schemata are the first dimensions of meaning at the interface between biology and culture, as such shared by all human beings, for the simple reason that all human beings have a body subject to the same fundamental biological laws. From this, it follows that these dimensions of meaning, even if exercised self-referentially by each subject, nonetheless operate as a *common semiotic plinth*, which guarantees a kind of common denominator for the coordination of action (which, as has been said previously, does not mean the capacity for targeting the action). Picking up on an example given earlier, quarreling is an emblematic example of how affective dimensions operate as a common semiotic plinth in the absence of any negotiated sharing. People do not need to agree to quarrel. Each disputant interprets the other's contingency in terms of an affective schema determined by the combination of three basic affective dimensions – |good/bad + powerful/weak/ + active/passive|. The affective schema of the disputants may vary – for example, the bully will configure the other as bad/passive/weak, while the victim will configure the other as bad/active/powerful – but such variations will still be within the perimeter of the variability of the intersubjective semiotic field underlying the coordination of the action of arguing. The ease with which one can fight even with perfect strangers testifies to how little prior agreement is needed to coordinate such action – just leave it to the visceral knowledge each of us has of the world. Paraphrasing Tolstoy, one could say that each subject uses low abstraction signs in their own way. All subjects use affective semiosis in the same way.

In this process of anchoring the intersubjective field to the semiotic plinth of affects, we grasp the role of simplification in grounding the social bond – in the beginning, there is not the logos, but affective semiosis; to it each subject returns as often as is needed to attune to the world, fueled by the transcendental confidence that, in the simplicity of meaning unfolding at that level, they will always find the form of the presence of the other. Elsewhere, one of us has metaphorized this process of compatibilization of the interpretive pluralism with the term *Pentecost effect* (Salvatore, 2016c). In the Acts of the Apostles (2:1–11), there is a story of how the Apostles, having received the Holy Spirit, preach to a crowd composed of people of different languages, and each one hears the speech as delivered in his own tongue. Here again, we set aside the religious significance of the narrative and focus on its metaphorical value – each hearer is locked in his own self-referential interpretive process (the tongue), from within which he assimilates the contingency of the other (he hears the Apostles' speech produced in his own language); in so doing, however, she/he participates in the collective construction of the action (the listening crowd). Therein lies the paradox of semiosis: the engine of intersubjectivity is an inherently self-referential mechanism.

All this leads to a conclusion: semiosis cannot fail – what it does is to move the compatibilization of the premise of sense to a level of greater abstraction, to the level of the semiotic plinth of affects. In this way, subjects keep themselves in dialogue by entertaining themselves around the few things that the unconscious talks about, as the Italian psychoanalyst Fornari (1979) puts it. From this point of view, the concept of failure of collusion (Carli, 1987a) should not be understood as an interruption of the collusive process. On the contrary, as the rampant forms of affectivization of the public sphere show, the greater the weakening of the complex devices of social regulation, the more the simplification of meaning is activated to anchor the coordination of action to the plinth of affective meaning (Salvatore et al., 2021, 2023). In this sense, in the presence of a destabilizing event, collusion does not fail; rather, it becomes even more disengaged from reality, in the sense that it feeds simplified forms of information – of the *Don't Look Up* type. What fails is evidently the ability to make the coordination of action consistent with the requirements of its targeting. What fails, in other words, is the ability to maintain the dialectical balance between the stability of the dynamic of sensemaking and the demand for adaptation that the environment presents to the subject.

The other side of the coin: semiotic innovation

In the previous section, we argued that the multiple manifestations of simplified forms of sensemaking reflect the self-referential nature of this dynamic, its conservative tendency, and the priority it gives to its own reproduction rather than exploring the variability of the environment. We have also highlighted the adaptive function of simplification, which is the foundation of social action. However, all this describes only part of the issue. One could say that it points to the mechanisms underlying the problems that the psychologist is called upon to address – subjects in many circumstances tend to cope with the variability of environmental states through interpretative simplifications that allow the dynamic of sensemaking to remain stable (see Chapter 2), albeit at the cost of a fall in its informational capacity. Ultimately, to paraphrase Freud, *the psychologist's clients suffer from (simplified) interpretations.*

The other side of the coin is the "invention of America." Human history and everyone's biography show how, in some circumstances, people and institutions are able to go beyond the Herculean columns of established premises and develop new languages and new meanings, giving up, at least partially and momentarily, the semiotic benefit offered by the Pentecost effect. In brief, the dynamic of sensemaking, the subjectivity it substantiates, is not condemned solely to simplifying – it is capable of innovation, too.

But what are the conditions that bring about innovation rather than semiotic simplification? What are the forms of social action that make possible ways of stabilizing the dynamic of sensemaking that result in interpretive legacies of increased complexity? Needless to add, this question is the crux of change theory, what connects it to the theory of the action – ultimately, psychological intervention finds its raison d'être in the activation of these kinds of forms of social action. To put it in an analogy, this questioning is similar to asking under what conditions gravity, instead of pushing toward the center of the earth, allows one to soar into the firmament.

Primary scenario

The answer to this question should be sought by retracing the distinction between the three types of semiotic change introduced in the previous paragraph. To each of them, we can correspond a form of action, which we call *primary scenario, secondary scenario,* and *intermediate scenario,* respectively.

As we have already noted, the extension of meanings (type 1 change; local variation) occurs when the premises of meaning are stable. We call *primary scenario* the action operating on the basis of stable premises of meaning that enables and fuels type 1 change. Lifeworlds (family relationships, friendship, and neighborhood relationships; on the concept of lifeworlds, elaborated in the context of phenomenological sociology, see Ardigò, 1982; for a psychological reading, see Cremaschi et al., 2021) are the paradigm of the primary scenario. These are domains of relationships founded on deeply rooted and shared premises of sense. The stability of the premises of sense underlying lifeworlds is linked to both a genetic and a structural factor. Genetically, the premises of sense active in lifeworlds emerge from shared participation in the social practices that substantiate such realms of relationship – individuals have been taught the same emotional dialect, one might say. There is, however, a structural feature that makes lifeworlds the context of stable dynamic of sensemaking – they have no product (Carli & Paniccia, 1999). In other words, lifeworlds are systems for the exercise of subjectivity, which, in themselves, have no other constraint than their own reproduction. A lifeworld is the exercise of the common bond substantiating the sense of self-experience and has no other reason for existence than its own existence. The love of a parent, the bond between two lovers, and friendship are ends in themselves. This, of course, does not mean that the relationships fueled by lifeworlds are void of constraints; such constraints, however, are exogenously imposed on the lifeworlds by their inscription within social systems – mafia, feuds, genocides, as well as the loss of interest in any other dimension of reality that blinds (usually momentarily) those in love, bear traces of the absolutizing tendency of the self-referentiality of lifeworlds. Moreover, the stability of the premises of sense that characterizes lifeworlds does not mean consensuality (see Chapter 2). On the contrary, lifeworlds are the sites of violent contrast between preferences, not infrequently resolved by resorting to violent acting out. One quarrels much more with those one loves than with those one is indifferent to. This is not at odds with our thesis of lifeworlds as the primary setting for the stability of premises of sense. In fact, as already noted, at the level of generalized signs, premises of sense are oppositional dimensions. What is shared is the dimension, not the polarity: if you like, one agrees on what it makes sense to dispute (being loved, the power to decide, the value of rank, etc.).

Secondary scenario

Type 2 change (infrastructural mutation) is transactional in nature. The subject is exposed to information that causes him or her to change the state of quality. The car previously considered very efficient is now interpreted as fairly or not very efficient. This means that the quality of the ground (in this case, the car as a functional device) remains unchanged while the state of the quality changes. We speak of negotiation in that to be type 2 change, it is necessary for the dynamic of sensemaking to be fueled by interpolation with a sequence of signs located in another region of the semiotic space. For example, various no-vaxers changed their minds when they found themselves in the intensive therapy unit grappling with the complications of COVID-19. In this case, the experience of illness (pain, prospect of death) and cure (relief related to the use of medical devices, experiences of doctors taking charge of the sick person) produced a shift in the trajectory of signs by which such subjects produce discourse around vaccination – a shift that manifested itself in signs such as "get vaccinated," "I was wrong," "vaccination is necessary," etc. In other cases, the sequence of interpolating signs has other subjects as its source – everyone changes their opinion as a result of the arguments offered by the interlocutor. The ability of interpolating signs to promote the migration of the trajectory of signs between regions of the semiotic field reflects the semiotic value of the signs at stake, i.e., the relationship between the associative force of such signs and their ability to channel the coordination of action. In other words, the more the social practice conveying interpolating signs remains stable, the more these signs operate as a semiotic attractor towards the subject, leading them to change their position in the semiotic field. From this point of view, the shift in position in the semiotic field that distinguishes type 2 change occurs in a similar way to how people learn a second language: by focusing on the context where it is spoken. The language signs produced in the context of use of that language are experienced by the subject as having high semiotic value, insofar as they allow action to become predictable in a progressively more effective way than the language signs of the mother tongue allow in that language context.

What has been said so far makes it possible to highlight an important aspect of the secondary scenarios within which type 2 changes take place – they are nonetheless based on compatibilized premises of sense. The subject in negotiation perceives interpolating signs as a possible form of experience insofar as such signs are nonetheless internal to the given range of variability – that is, such signs offer different versions of the state of quality that operates as a sense premise. To put it in functional terms, negotiation is a conflict that is exercised because of and on the basis of a shared framework. Buyer and seller may negotiate the price of buying and selling for a long time, but they can do so because they share the fundamental premise of sense about what a property is, what economic value is, the criteria that define each other's positions, etc. Similarly, a person who until recently considered a politician honest may find themselves changing that belief on the basis of information and discourse acquired in conversations and from media, which converge in pointing to the ethically questionable actions of the politician in question. In such a case, the interpolating signs may produce their effect in that they nonetheless remain within the |honesty| ground (which can assume many states, from fully honest to not at all honest).

It is worth pointing out that secondary scenarios are able to fuel negotiation because the type of action they substantiate is structurally different from that of primary scenarios. In the case of secondary scenarios, in fact, the action is product-oriented, which determines its foundation beyond itself. Secondary action finds its meaning in the realization of something that does not coincide with the reproduction of the action itself. The actors of a secondary scenario are not Beckettian characters restrained by dialogue: they interact to achieve a purpose, the representation of which operates as a superordinate regulator, at the core of the premise of sense in their relationship. It is this *triadic structure* that enables negotiation – without a purpose operating as the "third," interpolating signs would not be able to induce migration in the semiotic field, as they would be to a dyadic oppositional structure. In other words, the common prioritization of purpose allows actors to relativize the difference introduced by interpolating signs – namely, to treat it as a contingent event and thus utilize its informational content. Ultimately, the productive purpose operates as an invariant structure that enables and fuels variation. If the relationship between Tom and Dick saturates their exchange – i.e., if their relationship is set up as a primary scenario – any conflict introduced by the latter upon the signs produced by the former will be likened to a generalized negation: an offense, a betrayal, an attack. For example, Tom might tell Dick that the car the latter has purchased is of low quality. If what Tom sees of this act is only Dick's position toward himself, the criticism of the car will be interpreted as an attack directed at him. If, on the other hand, Tom takes the acquisition of information about the car and its functionality as the purpose of the discussion, namely, as an anchorage working as the "third," then the conflict introduced by Dick will remain contingent, functional to achieving the purpose. Incidentally, one of the main sources of criticality in institutions is the overflow of secondary scenarios into primary ones – i.e., the fact that organizational actors perceive themselves as interacting individuals rather than organizational functions governed by the structure of purposes (see in this regard the example of thanking the motorist who stops at the crosswalk; Section 5). A final clarification: the sharing of the purpose does not escape the Pentecost effect. Thus, here, it is not to say that participants in a secondary scenario give the same interpretation of the purpose; indeed, to foster the negotiation, it is enough for each actor to assume the action is constrained by an element working as the third. It does not matter what representation each driver gives of the red light – it is sufficient that their interpretations are compatible with the action of stopping the car.

Intermediate scenario

According to our thesis, type 3 change requires an additional type of catalyzer, which we will refer to in what follows as the *intermediate scenario*. In order to discuss its characteristics, it is opportune to take up what has already been observed about this type of change, that it consists of a modification of the constitutive quality of the ground. As mentioned, this modification comprehensively rewrites the premises of meaning; that is, the ground is redefined in its quality, not only in the state of quality, and this results in the reconfiguration of the object of experience itself. On the computational level, this corresponds to the fact that what changes is not the location of the subject within the given semiotic field – what we referred to earlier by the term "migration of the trajectory of signs" – but the structure of the semiotic field as such, more precisely its dimensionality (hence the definition of this change as structural transformation). This occurs as a result of the fact that the action generates a level of instability such that it cannot be managed through displacement in the given semiotic field, i.e., by merely changing the state of quality (infrastructural change). To the extent that instability exceeds this level – so to speak, to the extent it accesses an *over-threshold level* – the dynamic of sensemaking is induced to use the energy necessary for the structural transformation of the ground. Instability is dealt with in terms of accommodating the dimensionality of the semiotic space.

What has just been said outlines the two issues that need to be clarified: a) how does the action of the intermediate scenario produce over-threshold instability? and b) under what conditions does the dynamic of sensemaking handle over-threshold instability through increasing, rather than reducing, dimensionality?

The answer to the first question lies in recognizing that in the intermediate scenario, the premises of sense underlying the action are – at least potentially – violated in their entirety. Therein lies the difference with the secondary scenario. Indeed, in the secondary scenario, the violation of the premises does not involve the purpose of the action, which, therefore, operates as the instituted foundation of the negotiation. Let us return to the examples given previously. As noted, the possibility of changing one's mind about the functional quality of the car, the usefulness of the COVID-19 vaccine, or coming to an agreement on the purchase and sale of a property is based on stable premises of sense – the car as a functional means, the vaccine as a medical device, and the property as an economic good, respectively. On the basis of these compatibilized premises of sense, the actors are able to negotiate the varying states that these qualities may take – a vehicle may be more or less functional, a medical device may be more or less effective or more or less iatrogenic, and real estate may be given a range of economic values. Let us now imagine that the person who has been asked for an opinion on the car, the person who interacts with the no-vaxer, or the owner of the property respond to the interlocutor's proposal by saying, respectively, "the car is not only a means, it is also an aesthetic object. I will tell you what I think on this point"; "the question is not whether the vaccine is a way to protect you from COVID, the question is whether it is a resource to pursue a fundamental common good: the ability of the health care system to take charge of public health"; "do you think it is possible to put a price on the memories and emotions that this house means to me?" In all these cases, one is no longer negotiating – there is no longer a frame of purpose within which conflict is exercised between positions whose variability is kept internal to that shared premise of sense; rather, these three interlocutions introduce a radical violation of the premise of sense that underlies action. This violation ultimately consists of introducing a *stumbling block* in the reproduction of the Matthew effect (see Chapter 2, Section 6), that is, in the process by which the compatibilized premises make the object of experience a piece of reality. In sum, the global violation of the premises of sense does not involve a negotiating conflict about how to regulate the given action (as in the case of the secondary scenario) but radically transforms the landscape of the action. Where before there was discussion about the functionality of the car, now there is (or there could be) discussion about its aesthetics; where before there was discourse about the vaccine as a resource for the individual, now there is (or there could be) discourse about the vaccine as a way of pursuing the common good; where before there was an economic exchange now there is (or there could be) a claim to a relational good.

Ultimately, the intermediate scenario is *play*: an activity that absolutizes its premises for the pleasure of being able to violate them. Play is not fiction, but it is also not reality – it is the liminal space (Stenner, 2017; Salvatore & Venuleo, 2017) within which the reality of fiction (there is no play without the recognition of its separateness from other forms of action) and the fiction of reality (there is no fun if play is not taken seriously) pursue each other and refer to each other again and again. Here, we again see Bateson's (1972) observations on dolphins' play and its function of instantiating and, at the same time, de-absolutizing the aggressive gesture to operate as a performative affirmation of its negation.

Science (particularly scientific activity that has the pleasure/courage to play with its own assumptions) is an example of an intermediate scenario. Some artistic forms – for example, Magritte's logic-iconic games, Duchamp's conceptual elements, Piero Manzoni's provocations, and Banksy's performative objects offer themselves as further examples of intermediate scenario: texts that co-opt the interpreter in a continuous exercise of deconstruction of premises, to "imprison" her/him in an inexhaustible hermeneutic recursiveness.

Ultimately, the defining characteristic of the intermediate setting is its *recursiveness* – i.e., the fact that the action involves a function of suspending itself and revising the premises of sense placed at its foundation. This recursiveness can have different degrees of radicality due, on the one hand, to the *level of abstraction* and thus the degree of extension of the premises of sense subject to violation and, on the other hand, to the *temporal density* of this operation. From the first point of view, we can observe that the premise of sense can be located at the level of collections as well as at the levels of signs of higher generalization. The higher the level of abstraction, the deeper the destabilization introduced. To confine ourselves to one example among those proposed previously, if the property owner responded to the proposed purchase by questioning the very meaning of private property, the violation of the premise would evidently be at a higher level of abstraction than the violation introduced by anchoring the property to its relational value. From the point of view of temporal density, the alternation between the exercise of premises and their violation can follow more or less intense cycles, forming a continuum. At one extreme, there is the *weak* intermediate scenario, in which the violation of premises occurs as a discrete event that operates as a parenthesis within the normal flow of action, allowing the latter to access levels of greater complexity progressively; at the other extreme, there is the *strong* intermediate scenario, characterized by continuous recursiveness, where the exercise of the action tends asymptotically to overlap with the violation of premises. In the strong intermediate scenario, then, action is both the vector and the object of systematic deconstruction of the semiotic conditions of its own operation. In terms of dynamic systems theory, in the strong intermediate scenario, the production of instability is its metastable equilibrium. The psychoanalytic setting is the paradigmatic example of the strong intermediate scenario. As an ideal model, such a setting pursues a methodological goal of suspending action (Carli, 1987b): it is an action that proposes, recursively, to analyze – therefore to violate – the subjective and intersubjective conditions (= the premises of sense) that underlie it. The psychoanalytic setting has no goals other than its own reproduction over time to analyze the condition (i.e., the instituted premises of sense) of such reproduction. This, of course, does not mean that it cannot produce utility for those who participate in it. However, such utility does not regulate the action – it is a kind of side effect (for a discussion of analysis as a recursive methodological exercise without memory and desire, see, for example, Sandler & Dreher, 1996).

We class as intermediate the scenario that induces type 3 change because it is a mixture of primary and secondary scenarios. As we have observed, the intermediate scenario shares with the secondary scenario the rule of violation of the premises of sense. At the same time, the intermediate scenario radicalizes this violation exercise of premises. On the other hand, this means that in the intermediate scenario, there is no external purpose grounding the action: the intermediate scenario is reproduced as a systematic exercise of rewriting itself. From this point of view, the actors in an intermediate scenario are also restrained by dialogue, as in the case of the primary scenario; however, a particular dialogue conveys the systematic deconstruction of its own premises.

These considerations bring us to the second question: what conditions allow the intermediate scenario to fuel the complexification of the semiotic field rather than its simplification – increasing rather than reducing dimensionality? Other things being equal, as mentioned previously, simplifying is a mode that requires less energy expenditure.

Our thesis is as follows: the violation of the premises of sense exposes the subject to additional dimensions of environmental variability, namely, those dimensions that the premises kept inert in the background. Now, to the extent that the intermediate scenario makes available signs that activate new dimensions of meaning – hereafter: *source signs*, the subject can introduce such dimensions into the semiotic field without incurring an excess in the expenditure of energy with respect to the "downward" mapping played out in reducing the dimensionality of the semiotic field. In the previous examples, if the source signs proposed by the interlocutor – the car as an aesthetic object, the vaccine as a contribution to the common good, and real estate as a place of relations – are already present in the cultural milieu of the subject exposed to the violation of the premises, the adoption of such signs will require an expenditure of energy no different from that associated with dealing with the violation in terms of dimensionality reduction.

It should be added that the possibility of mobilizing source signs does not depend on their potential availability only. Such signs are mobilized to the extent that they are in the intermediate scenario as part of its implicit procedural knowledge. This means that psychological intervention cannot be limited to making source signs available; it is also necessary to root such signs within the intersubjective field of intervention so that their potential availability can be translated into an actual ability to mobilize them. For example, for patient Mr. D. (see Section 4), the therapist's interventions aimed at activating the interpretation of the marital relationship as |patient-gives/wife-receives| constitute a cluster of source signs that activate the give/receive dimension of the semiotic field. It is not enough, however, for the therapist to produce utterances related to such types of signs; it is necessary for them to become progressively rooted in the clinical exchange, becoming an integral part of the semiotic device that governs such action. This is not unlike what happens in language learning, where it is not enough to read about the representation of semantics and syntax in books; using them is necessary so that they can be progressively assimilated in terms of procedural memories.

4

THEORY OF THE ACTION

This chapter is devoted to the theory of the action, the part of GTPI that focuses on the regulation of intervention, i.e., the criteria and tools through which to activate, foster, and orient the catalyzers of change examined in the previous chapter. Consistent with the approach of the entire volume, the discussion in what follows will be kept on a general and abstract level – the only one that can encompass the many forms of professional psychological action. As presented in this chapter, the theory of the action is thus not designed to enrich the reader's technical background with procedural and operative suggestions; rather, it is intended to define a general methodological framework that offers, precisely by virtue of its abstraction, a conceptual basis for the techniques and tools used in the various domains of intervention.

The chapter is divided into three parts. In the first, a typology of intervention vectors is proposed. Each vector is a specific function that the psychologist can exercise to activate catalyzers of change. In the second, some general criteria that qualify the way of targeting the use of vectors are explored – in particular, the semiotic conception of the setting, the organized structure of the intervention, and the forms of reporting and analysis of results. The third section is devoted to abduction, proposed here as a fundamental mode of knowledge production used by the intervention.

1 Vectors of intervention

This section is devoted to presenting a typology of the ways in which intervention promotes change. We call these ways vectors to highlight the idea of professional action as a vehicle for modes of social exchange capable of generating semiotic innovation through the activation of its catalyzers. The typology is

DOI: 10.4324/9781003449362-5

a reworking of the schema proposed by Salvatore (2016a), developed using the distinction between the three types of changes/scenarios introduced in Chapter 3. Before proceeding, a general caveat. The proposed typology is not about operative procedures; rather, it concerns functions, the realization of which requires operative modes that vary from context to context. Different vectors can be realized through similar modes of operation; what distinguishes them is the purpose for which those modes are used. In other words, the link between the vector and its function is not invariant. Meaning, as mentioned previously (see Chapter 2), depends on the sign it follows; consequently, the result of the vector is not inherent to it: it depends on how it is interpreted in context. More generally, this means that psychologists do not assume that the meaning of their actions corresponds to what they attribute to it. That meaning, in fact, is always produced through the interaction with the client's interpretive activity. This makes a conceptual and methodological apparatus of criteria quite useful since only by reference to it is the psychologist in a position to reconstruct – always a posteriori and often following a demanding course of analysis and reflection on their own actions – the meaning that their action has acquired, in and because of the intersubjective field with the client.

Primary scenario vectors. The enhancement of meaning

This cluster covers the functions of the psychologist that promote local variation (see Chapter 3) in the meaning (knowledge, beliefs, information packets) already held by the client system so as to consolidate it. Such enhancement can take different forms – for example, expansion of the objects referred to, differentiation, and assimilation of additional elements. Each of these forms lends itself to being associated with one or more vectors, some of which, without claiming to be exhaustive, are recalled in what follows.

Validation. This vector is aimed at consolidating the client's meaning through the legitimacy that can be derived from the consensus that the psychologist, in his role of expert, expresses about it. Consider, for example, a client who exposes to the psychologist the reasons behind a decision he has just made and the psychologist who, in response, informs him that she/he finds those reasons soundness and agreeable.

Specification. This vector recalls what in the psychoanalytic theory of technique is called clarification – a reformulation of what the patient proposes aimed at making her/his communication more comprehensible and coherent (Langs, 1973/1974). This operation can be applied in virtually any intervention situation. Consider the following situation. A politician meets with a psychologist to develop a communication strategy aimed at increasing support for his/her political party. The politician recalls various circumstances of people of different ages and social backgrounds who have expressed negative opinions about the party for which he/she works. After listening to this, the psychologist says, "If I understand correctly, by referring to these episodes, you mean to signal to me that, in your opinion, your political party is undergoing a general erosion of support." We consider this an example of clarification because, in this case, the operation performed by the psychologist is to organize the meaning communicated by the client into a more efficient form – in this case, into a more synthetic and abstract representation.

Schematization. To schematize a meaning is to represent it in terms of the significant relationships that substantiate it (Valsiner, 2020). The conceptual map is an example of schematization: the representation of a package of knowledge related to an object in terms of a network of logical-semantic and/or functional relationships among elements. We consider schematization to be a form of meaning enhancement in that, similarly to specification, it does not change the meaning held by the client; on the contrary, by allowing the latter to be represented in terms of its essential structure, it promotes its stabilization.

Making explicit. We group here the set of diverse operations by which the client is enabled to represent in declarative form a meaning otherwise operating at the implicit level. Implicit is not intended here to be synonymous with latent. Implicit meaning is the body of knowledge accessible to those participating in the communication, which is not stated because it is considered already shared by communication participants (Sbisà, 2002). For example, stating, "John did not take the bus because he had no way to get a ticket," gives the implicit meaning that to take the bus, one needs to hold a ticket. Latent meaning, on the other hand, is the meaning that operates as the premise of sense underlying the interpretability of what is heard, thought, said, or done. In the terms proposed earlier (see Chapter 2), implicit meaning is a form of *significance in praesentia*, and latent meaning of *significance in absentia*. The following is an example of explicitness. In a training meeting with the sales staff of a software company, several participants, invited to propose critical situations worthy of analysis, report events that, although diverse, present as a problem the situation of a customer expressing dissatisfaction with the company. The consultant, after having collected the various proposals, points out that they imply the idea that the customer's satisfaction is a priority value.

Enrichment. By this term, we mean to denote the vector aimed at allowing the client access to semiotic resources that, precisely, enrich the client's system of meanings. The new information may be used by the client to validate a belief or expand/limit its scope of application; in other cases, the additional information is what enables the client to make a choice among the alternatives available. One of us has recently been serving as an advisor of a public health service engaged with anti-gambling interventions (more details on the case in Chapter 6). The service in question operates on the basis of a community intervention model: it takes into consideration as a determinant of gambling behavior not only the intrapsychic characteristics of individual gamblers but also the ways gambling is interpreted and socially regulated within the community and interpersonal networks. Part of the consultancy was devoted to testing this model empirically on the territorial area of interest. The results produced by the research carried out for this purpose are, among other things, an example of information enrichment. More precisely, these results allowed the client to validate its intervention model, to extend its application to several additional actors mediating the relationship between gamers and social networks (e.g., bet room operators) and make some choices about the targets of intervention.

Assimilation. With this term, we refer to the psychologist's actions aimed at supporting the client in the use of their own system of meanings. Through this operation, the psychologist aims to improve the client's ability to use the semiotic resources available to them to make sense of the aspects of reality with which they relate. In this case, the client produces new meaning (the interpretation of the aspect of reality); however, they do so from within the given system of meaning, assimilating the aspect of reality to it. In doing so, the given system of meaning is enhanced through the very possibility of exercising it on a new element of experience. One example of the exercise of this vector is when in a group discussion – for example, in a training context – the psychologist prompts and supports participants to analyze a situation of interest from their point of view.

Secondary scenario vectors. The didacticization of meaning

We collect in this cluster the vectors through which the psychologist introduces an element of conflict with respect to the client's interpretive activity so as to solicit the latter to accommodate – that is, to make an infrastructural modification of their own system meaning. As we have had occasion to point out (see Chapter 3, Section 5), the conflict that fuels negotiation is local rather than structural: it does not affect the system of meaning globally, but one specific aspect of it – the state of the quality comprising the ground, rather than the quality as such.

Activation. By this term, we mean the vector by which the psychologist fosters the salience of the client's semiotic resource (a belief, a knowledge package). The resource is already present in the client's system of meaning; however, we consider this type of operation a negotiating vector rather than a reinforcing one (i.e., a primary scenario vector) because its purpose is to solicit a modification of the system of meaning – more precisely, a modification that is not about content but about the underlying hierarchy of preferences. One way of pursuing activation is to reinforce – emphasizing its value, proposing a generalization – the meaning the client produces (e.g., by expressing an opinion) so as to make it assume centrality in the subsequent development of the communication. For example, during the meeting with the psychologist, a participant proposes a parallel between the conflict that had arisen with the user and the conflict present within the work team. The psychologist takes the ball and says, "You are making a suggestion that deserves to be explored further. You are saying that there may be a connection between what happens at the level of the service life and what happens with the users. This hypothesis outlines a line of exploration that is worth pursuing." The psychologist has thus operated a clarification – he rephrases what the client said so as to systematize it; in this way, he lays the foundation for valorizing it through its generalization and proposal of using it as anchorage of the subsequent activity of analysis.

Deactivation. This is the opposite vector to the previous one. In this case, the psychologist works to reduce the salience of a client's semiotic resource to make it lose relevance as the organizer of their interpretive activity. For example, in the context of an interview, resource development managers dwell on comments and observations focused on the personality traits of employees. After listening to them for a sufficiently long time, the psychologist proposes, as the next step in the discussion, to shift the focus from people's personalities to the functions their roles fulfill in the company.

Differentiation. This vector is aimed at restricting the use of a semiotic resource by placing a limit on the contexts within which it can frame the interpretation of experience. Differentiation is thus similar to deactivation in that both operate in the sense of placing constraints on the client's interpretive activity. The difference between these two operations lies in this: while in the case of deactivation, the constraint concerns the semiotic resource, in the case of differentiation, the constraint concerns the object (the domain of reality) on which the semiotic resource is exercised. For example, in a training job aimed at computer technicians of a software company, the psychologist pointed out the tendency of the trainees to think of the company's customers as if they were fellow computer scientists evaluating the products they made with standards, expectations, and technical skills equivalent to their own. In doing so, the psychologist worked to limit the extension of the meaning used by technicians to make sense of their professional activity to the company's customers.

Relativization. This vector is intended to highlight the contingent quality of the meaning produced – the fact that it is always and, in any case, contextual, linked to the modes of the action it helps to regulate, an expression of the point of view in terms of which the subject's participation in the action is configured. Thus, this function does not address the content; rather, it allows for a subjective appropriation of meaning on the part of the client, that is, the possibility of recognizing it as something that speaks of the subject who produced it rather than being a mere mirror of the facts of reality. At the same time, the recognition of the partiality and contingency of the meaning produced creates the conditions for recognizing the presence of other points of view, thus valuing the plurality of positions as a source of enrichment of the interpretation of experience. The technique of role reversal, often used in psychosocial counseling, is an example of relativization. Group participants are asked to initiate a role-play in which they assume what, in reality, is the role of the interlocutor/alter – for example, the physician plays the role of the patient. This puts the participant in a position to enter the logic of the other and, in so doing to, recognize how the same reality can be interpreted from a plurality of perspectives, such that each observation tells more about the observer than the observed (Maturana & Varela, 1980).

Confutation. By this term, we mean the psychologist's action aimed at pointing out the inconsistencies present within the client's discourse. This is done to reduce the tendency of such discourse to reproduce itself self-referentially, that is, to find within itself the reasons for its own validity. Inconsistencies can be of different kinds: it may concern the logical relationship between parts of the discourse, for example, affirming something and at the same time its opposite; the functional aspect, for example, speaking of an initiative as aiming at certain purposes and at the same time not including in it the essential roles and resources for pursuing them; the pragmatic aspect, for example, dwelling on secondary topics in a meeting with the result of leaving little time for the important points of the agenda. Consider the following episode that occurred to one of us in the context of an initial meeting with a high school principal who had requested advice on designing an intervention addressing the school's students and designed to reduce dropout rates. For a good half hour, the headmistress expressed to the psychologist her concerns about teachers, criticized for their lack of motivation, tendency to disengage, and unwillingness to collaborate with the school and colleagues. The psychologist, after listening, observed, "From the way you are talking, it would seem that the intervention you are requesting should be aimed at the teachers rather than the students."

Falsification. Like confutation, this vector aims to subject the meaning produced by the client to criticism. In this case, however, the criticism is not intended to point out internal inconsistencies in the discourse but the conflict between the statements and the data. In many cases, research performed in the context of intervention is used (also) to this end. Recently, one of us, with others, conducted a community study aimed at surveying attitudes toward goods confiscated from organized crime (see Chapter 6 for details). The research, commissioned by a regional administration in Southern Italy, showed that attitudes toward confiscated goods – and thus the propensity to valorize them socially and economically – reflected the perception of institutions and the trust placed in them. This result made it possible to challenge the idea, widespread among those responsible for promoting the community use of the confiscated goods, that the low social valorization of confiscated property depended on economic, functional, and management factors only.

Analogical projection. This vector dialectizes the client's meaning by establishing an analogy with a similar social context, which could highlight the limit on the validity of the client's meaning. One of us uses this feature with psychology students to highlight their propensity to express hypotheses and analysis in subjective terms, as a form of personal opinion, expressed without any anchorage to constructs and/or data – for example, with locutions such as "it comes to mind that . . ., " "I believe that . . ., " or "my opinion is . . ." In some cases, the comment offered in response to this mode of expression is along the lines of: "Imagine a doctor, whom you have approached for a diagnostic opinion about some symptoms that are bothering you, responding, 'it comes to mind that you have . . .'. Or, imagine an engineer stating, 'The way I feel it, the cottage I'm designing for her will stand.' What would your reaction be? Would you recommend this professional to a friend?" The analogical projection here is between two contexts – the professional context of the psychologist (as the practice foreshadowed by the psychology student's discourses) and that of other professional figures. The fact that both contexts belong to the same domain (the profession) allows the projection. What is projected is the subjective form of the language; in this way, the limit of validity, and more generally, the meaning underlying subjective utterances is highlighted in its being an act of signification that deserves to be subject to critical scrutiny and/or analysis of its own premise of sense.

Negotiation. The specificity of this vector lies in the fact that, unlike the previous ones, in this case, the psychologist antagonizes the client's system of meaning through the fielding of an alternative meaning. Thus, he does not merely act, so to speak, as a dialectical sideliner to the client's interpretive activity; he proposes an alternative meaning with which the client must come to terms and negotiate precisely. The psychologist can introduce the alternative meaning either in declarative terms, i.e., through a symbolic representation or in performative terms, as part of the form of the action exercised. A few years ago, one of us contributed to the drafting of a paper of the Italian Psychology Association explicitly critical of the immigration policies of the Italian government of the time. Based on a wealth of theoretical and empirical literature, the paper (Italian Association of Psychology, 2019) argues that forms of defensive reactivity and closure with respect to otherness once mobilized in the social system, do not merely inform attitudes toward the outgroup – in this case, toward immigrants; rather, they inevitably end up contaminating the quality of the relations inside the ingroup as well. Fostering such forms, therefore, paradoxically backfires against the goals of social cohesion that anti-immigration measures claim to pursue. As can be seen, such a document is a form of negotiation: an alternative meaning conveyed through language – the government believes its migration policy is effective; the psychologist claims, in contrast, that it is iatrogenic. An example of performative negotiation, on the other hand, is the following: some time ago, a school headmistress asked one of us to meet with a class, one of whose members had a few days earlier died as a result of a tragic accident that occurred during school hours. By doing so, the headmistress thought she could help the students process the trauma of seeing their classmate die before their eyes due to an absurd fatality. The psychologist understood that the density of emotions that saturated the entire intersubjective field of school life at that moment would leave no room for negotiation of a symbolic nature conveyed by words. He then merely proposed that the meeting with the students be preceded by a meeting with the teachers, from whom would be collected information regarding the students' state. The purpose of this proposal was not functional in nature – it was rather the performative way of conveying the meaning: |the teachers are those whose function it is to help students to elaborate the traumatic experience, and to do so, they must be supported in their ability to make sense of the intersubjective field of school life|. Incidentally, the meeting with the teachers was sufficient: the psychologist did not need to meet with the students – it was the teachers who took over the function of taking charge of both their traumatic experience and that of the students.

Intermediate scenario vectors. The deconstruction of meaning

We report in what follows some vectors that are aimed at fostering the deconstruction of meaning – that is, the reflection on the premises of sense underlying the client's interpretative activity. Deconstruction of meaning is not analogous to critical analysis and negotiation of meanings. Deconstruction addresses the *significance in absentia* rather than the *significance in praesentia*; moreover, and most importantly, it does not operate from a normative perspective: it does not make evaluations of merit (of a functional kind, of logical coherence, of conformity with data); on the contrary, it suspends judgment, operating – as Bion puts it – without memory and without desire. Subjectively, the proposed deconstruction/reflection is often experienced similarly to how one reacts to criticism. This is because deconstruction induces a (local) interruption of the client's ability to generate meaning. Deconstruction, however, is not critical analysis: in the case of criticism, the meaning is dialectized – and this is done through meaning that is compatible with the premises of sense underpinning the criticism – in the case of deconstruction, the meaning is suspended. To use an image, the negotiating psychologist stands to the tennis player whose strokes force the opponent into certain movements, just as the deconstructing psychologist stands to the tennis player who stops playing in order to discuss with the other tennis player the tactics of play used. We consider the difference between critique and deconstruction central to psychological intervention. Accordingly, we will use the two terms – analysis and deconstruction (in some cases, we will use the term *reflection*, in its psychoanalytic sense, as a synonym of deconstruction) – differently so that it is clear what kind of scenario/change is being referred to. Incidentally, the rigor in the use of psychological language is, in our opinion, one of the essential conditions for promoting the development of the scientific-professional system. Psychology will not get very far if psychologists continue to use terms such as *reflection* – as well as *affect, desire, motivation*, etc. – in a polysemous way, similar to how we may do in daily life when we produce statements such as "I've thought it over, I'll have cappuccino rather than coffee," "after careful reflection, I realized I was wrong," and "think carefully before you answer!"

Interpretation. We use this term to denote the vector aimed at making the client's premises of sense representable, hence an object of discourse. Historically, in the field of psychology, interpretation is associated with the theory of psychoanalytic technique, where it is understood in a plurality of ways, in a general sense referring to the unraveling of unconscious meaning conveyed by the subject's communication (Freud, 1899/1953; see also, for example, Etchegoyen, 2005; Fornari, 1983; Langs, 1973/1974). The function of interpretation, however, has a broader field of use, ultimately coinciding with the totality of human signification – wherever there is a text, it can be the object of interpretation, i.e., analyzed in the premises on which it is based. This generalized definition allows us to return to what was said in the introduction of this section and further clarify what interpretation *is not*: it is not the search for the "hidden cause" of which the client's text is the effect; it is not the discovery of the latent purpose that drives the client (on the discussion of the use of efficient and final cause view in psychological intervention, see Chapter 1); just as it is not the understanding of what the client "really wants to say." As we are conceptualizing it here, the interpretive vector is the exercise of identifying the ground – namely, the premises of sense – by reason of which the text subjected to interpretation acquires meaning. Underlying this definition is the idea (see Chapter 2) that any combination of signs, any text, to be construed, must be based on a meaning of a higher level of generalization, operating as a premise of sense – and acquires meaning by reason of it. Interpretation aims to abductively identify (see Section 3) such generalized meaning, which operates ultimately as a *condition of the text's thinkability* – that is, a condition that, if assumed, endows the text with meaning. It comes back in this regard to what a distinguished cultural psychologist (Shweder, 1991) said about his discipline, whose function, according to him, is to identify the system of beliefs and values by reason of which behaviors and thought forms of other societies, at first sight incomprehensible, sometimes in profound contrast to Western values, become sound, rational – one of the examples given by the author is Sati, the practice of having a widow burn alive on her husband's funeral pyre. Interpretation follows the same logic – it is ultimately a *function of humanizing otherness*: the search for meaning that makes the gesture/discourse human that otherwise, if interpreted from the interpreter's premises of sense, would appear radically other. Interpretation thus challenges those who practice it profoundly – it requires the interpreter to overlook their own premises of sense in order to create the semiotic room where the conditions of thinkability of what is being interpreted can be constructed. An example of interpretation conveyed by an empirical model is the one presented in Chapter 2 (Figure 2.2), where the symbolic universes active within the cultural milieu of a set of European countries were shown. As we noted there, each symbolic universe can be considered a premise of sense at the foundation of a segment of the population's beliefs and opinions about the future, interpersonal relationships, institutions, etc. In turn, symbolic universes can be interpreted as generalized signs inscribed in even more generalized latent dimensions of meaning, the interweaving of which generates the semiotic field that substantiates the cultural milieu.

Performative structuring. This vector is based on the recognition of the mutual inherence of signification and action (see Chapter 2): sensemaking is the shape of social action, and social action is the way sensemaking is instantiated. This means that at the abstract level of general theory, sensemaking and action are the same – similarly to what happens between heat and movement of molecules. On a level closer to experience, however, sensemaking and action are distinguishable – on this level, we will therefore say that the two terms are connected by a bond of mutual influence: the forms of thought configure the forms of action, and vice versa.

Let us return to the case of Mr. D., presented in Chapter 3. In the light of the discussion presented here, the therapist's interventions aimed at activating an additional dimension of the semiotic field (giving/receiving) are examples of performative structuring – the therapist performs an action that determines an environment whose regulation by the patient requires making the new dimension of meaning salient. Structuring can operate in a multiplicity of ways. The aspects of the intervention on which it can act are innumerable – from those related to logistics (e.g., the arrangement of chairs, the presence of notepads for note-taking) to temporal ones (the strictness of adherence to time, the duration of meetings, their frequency), from organizational ones (the forms and channels of communication, the decision about who participates in meetings; who summons whom) to pragmatic ones (calling each other by name or not, the manner of taking turns in conversation). All these elements have, as is obvious, a functional valence; however, they also have a semiotic-performative valence: they are vectors of intersubjective fields of meaning, which contribute significantly to shaping the interpretation of the context – for example, as a context of interpersonal relations centered on identity or as a context governed by the value of competence and responsibility over outcome.

To summarize

The scheme of vectors presented in this section can be read as a list of points or in temporal terms. As a list, the scheme proposes a set of possible vectors to which the psychologist can refer. In temporal terms, the vectors are an indication of the various phases of which the intervention can be composed. This does not mean that all interventions will comprise and follow the trajectory of the three proposed clusters; local conditions will determine which combination of vectors is appropriate to use.

The first cluster of vectors is characterized by their function of consolidating the meaning given. These vectors address the *significance in praesentia* and aim to strengthen it. The term consolidate is to be understood in two different ways: 1) to consolidate, in the context of the relationship, the representation of the object being dealt with (agreement on the object of discourse); and 2) to consolidate the meaning ascribed by the client to the events in which they are involved. The first function of the term consolidate (1) is to extract a possible order from the set of discourse elements. Imagine the client's request as the depositing of many elements on a table and the psychologist as the one who tries to extract order from what often appears confusing (unknown, newly encountered). Such order is necessarily an interpretive act in the sense that it extracts one configuration among many possible ones. For this purpose, the psychologist may use the vector of *clarification*, that is, identifying a summary meaning of the objects placed on the table (say, fruit) or a *schematization*, which highlights the relationship between the objects or, again, he or she may *make the implicit explicit*, by taking the class that, from the client's point of view, collects the elements on the table in a meaningful order, as the object of the discourse shared with the client. The goal is always the same (sharing the object of discourse), while different contextual conditions will suggest what order to give the items. By the second meaning of consolidate (2), we refer, for example, to the possibility of *validating* the meaning that has previously been shared or the possibility of *enriching* it or, again, the possibility of *assimilating* other aspects of experience to it.

The second cluster covers vectors aimed at *dialectizing meaning*. Again, these vectors refer to the *significance in praesetia* expressed by the client, yet this significance is addressed with the aim of modifying them on the level of their content. Note that such modification is not without costs and requires adequate time and mode to be elaborated. The psychologist may act to modify the meaning – for example, a belief – held by the client by focusing on an otherwise marginal aspect (*activation*) or, conversely, by *deactivating* a meaning assumed to be central by the client. Again, the psychologist may reduce the set of objects to which the belief refers (*differentiation*) or encourage recognition of how what the client believes to be true is an expression of one of the viewpoints involved (*relativization*). Again, the psychologist may press the client to grasp the inconsistencies (at various levels) internal to their discourse (*confutation*) or the contradiction between the meaning expressed and the context (*falsification* and *analogical projection*). Finally, the psychologist may *negotiate* with the client a different meaning from that proposed by the client. It is worth adding that, though we grouped them together because of their common function, these vectors operate with different process conditions. *Activation*, for example, is quite different from *negotiation*. The latter requires a much stronger consolidation of the working relationship with the client than is required by the use of the former.

The third cluster of vectors aims to reorganize the premises of sense at the foundation of the client's interpretative activity. It thus addresses *significance in absentia*. The purpose of these vectors is to promote the development of the client's point of view rather than a modification of its outcome. This purpose can be pursued through speech-mediated actions – what we have termed *interpretation* – or in performative terms – what we have termed *performative structuring*.

2 General principles and devices of the intervention

This section is devoted to a discussion of some general principles and devices that qualify the ways in which intervention vectors are used. In particular, we will consider the following aspects: the setting, the organizational structure of the intervention, and the ways in which professional action is reported and its outcomes are validated.

The setting

In what follows, we propose a definition of the intervention setting derived from the semiotic theory adopted in this volume. From the perspective of that theory, the *setting is the premise of sense in terms of which the intervention is constituted in the psychologist's mind* (Salvatore, 2016a). This means that the setting is not the set of material, normative, and functional features activated by the intervention and regulative of the relationship between psychologist and client system – e.g., schedule, time, fee, logistics, etc. Rather, it is the *significance in absentia* that leads to the selection of the objects of the intervention from the infinite possibilities of selection offered by the intersubjective field in which the relationship between psychologist and client system unfolds and the criteria in terms of which these objects are treated – e.g., the vectors described previously. In sum, the setting is not a state/entity; rather, it is the psychologist's interpretive process, which determines the conditions of the professional actions: the lens through which the psychologist "filters" the experience of participation in the intersubjective field of the relationship with the client system and, in so doing, makes the intervention emerge as a thinkable object of experience. In other words, the setting is the meta-interpretive rule that generates the intervention as a peculiar semiotic micro-universe. Psychological intervention in this is like Monopoly – a rule that leads to stabilizing interpretations of signs, transforming them into a world inhabited by events and entities (houses, hotels, bills, prisons, Virginia Avenue, etc.). Consider any relationship between a psychologist and a client. What *exists* is the intersubjective field activated by the two subjects. Such a field can be filtered in an infinite number of ways: as a conversation between friends, as a power conflict, as a helping relationship, etc. Such a field *becomes* intervention to the extent that the setting extracts such a form from it – that is, to the extent that the ground made relevant is that of the exchange between a client and a professional psychologist aimed at a given purpose.

This semiotic conception of the setting does not deny the value of the material and concrete aspects that mediate and convey the intervention. Consistent with the psycho-semiotic conception discussed in the previous chapters, it considers these elements as *artifacts* (see Chapter 3), that is, signs crystallized in reified forms that, like any other kind of sign, generate meaning because of the premises at the basis of their use.

A major implication of the semiotic conception of setting is that, by definition, *intervention is constituted in terms that are autonomous from common sense*. In other words, intervention is a game that follows its own rules, different, in some cases even counterintuitively, from those that preside over the definition of the social settings of everyday life (Salvatore & Valsiner, 2014). The data that the psychologist processes within the intervention context are not those that the client "sees" with the eyes of common sense; they are those that the psychologist constitutes as a result of "filtering" the intersubjective field by means of the setting. This, of course, does not mean that the intervention setting alone is able to lay the foundation of the relationship with the client, similar to Baron Münchhausen's lifting himself up by his pigtail. In fact, every intervention moves on two levels. On the one hand, the psychologist elaborates the intersubjective field of social action through the premises of sense defined by the psychological setting; on the other hand, the intersubjective field comes to be determined by the fact that psychologist and client share a common system of instituted premises that are placed at the foundation of the class of social actions to which, according to the society's point of view, the psychologist's performance belongs, such as the canons that make the relationship between psychologist and client a form of professional service, operating as purposeful action, regulated by public norms, characterized by transactions and goals having economic counter-value. None of these canons are intrinsic features of the psychological intervention; rather, they are historically and culturally instituted meanings that, given their unreflective and stable nature (Harmon, 2020), have acquired the status of facts for the social actors who take them as the foundation of their interaction. Ultimately, this means that the intervention is fueled by a constant dialectic between two semiotic attractors – the practical knowledge of everyday social life, which determines the very conditions of the encounter between psychologist and client, and the psychological setting, continually called upon, like Sisyphus, to reconfigure the meaning of what happens because of the scientific categories placed at the foundation of the intervention (Salvatore, 2016a). We speak of dialectics for this reason: the two attractors are intrinsically in conflict with each other, and at the same time, each is constituted as a condition of existence of the other: there would be no possibility of exercising the psychological setting if common sense did not provide the semiotic conditions for the encounter between psychologist and client; there would be no possibility of such an encounter if it did not present itself as the object of the reconfiguration of meaning operated by the setting. To use an example: the client who goes to the psychologist does so on the basis of the commonsensical interpretation of his or her own problems and of the psychologist's function (we will return to this point in the next chapter) as well as of the established meanings that define the respective roles of professional and client. The psychologist does not deny this attractor of meaning; at the same time, he does not assume it as the foundation of the intervention relationship – on the contrary, he considers it recursively as a continuous starting point of the development of the psychological setting through which the goals, functions, and data of the intervention are constituted.

Intervention as organization

Intervention is a social action that mobilizes relational and material devices with the aim of bringing about conditions useful for activating, fostering, and orienting the catalyzers of change discussed in the previous chapter. This means that the *intervention is an organization, and as such, it must be designed, exerted, and analyzed*: a system that equips itself with constraints in order to remain goal-oriented. Like any other organization, the intervention is characterized by roles, functions, areas of responsibility, ways of decision-making, management and control, information exchange, horizontal integration of processes, and management of critical events.

As a matter of course, specific forms and contents of the organization of intervention differ because of the areas of professional action. A clinical intervention aimed at the individual implies a very different organization from that required by a corporate training or community development intervention. However, it is possible to recall, without presuming to be exhaustive, some parameters that deserve to be considered in both the design and management of the intervention.

First, every intervention implies a *distribution of functions among the actors involved*: psychologist, client, and stakeholders. Distributing functions means establishing who takes responsibility for what. The distribution is all the more differentiated, the greater the articulation of the intervention and the higher the number of actors involved: the distribution of functions between the psychologist working at his private practice as a psychotherapist and his client is obviously simpler than that involved in an intervention involving a team engaged in an intervention at a plurality of locations in a medium-sized company. The functions that need to be defined in their distribution are both those of operative nature (*line*, according to the terminology of management theory), that is, the set of operations through which the change that the intervention sets out to achieve is pursued, and those of a service nature (*staff*), that is, the set of operations that perform the task of ensuring the resources (human, organizational, economic, symbolic) necessary for the intervention to be carried out in a manner consistent with the purpose pursued.

As is obvious, the psychologist's contribution to the operational function is central; this does not detract from the fact that the client also contributes to the fulfillment of this type of function. Think of the members of a team operating within a community health service who benefit from advice and who a) design with the consultant psychologist action research aimed at analyzing their way of operating in relation to the context to enhance its appropriateness and effectiveness, and b) interpret results of the research in discussion with the consultant, to translate them into criteria and development objectives for their own work. In doing so, team members are exercising an operational function, which contributes to the pursuit of the purpose of the intervention. The distribution of responsibilities concerning service functions is an important aspect of intervention. Many of the operations that fall under this umbrella are often left in the realm of the implicit, distributed according to commonsensical criteria that belong to the practical knowledge of people and social groups. For example, when a person asks for an appointment with a clinical psychologist, both take it for granted that they will meet at the latter's office – i.e., they assume, as a matter of course, that the function of arranging logistical resources is under the psychologist's responsibility. Service functions, depending on contexts and circumstances, may need to be made explicit and subject to agreement. For example, in various interventions involving members of the client organization, the presence of incentives for participation in the intervention is a sensitive point on which the psychologist and client should agree.

Second, each intervention involves a *logical and temporal articulation*. In many cases, the intervention implies the need to organize the different operations into clusters functionally connected to each other, i.e., defining which results are to be produced first to act as conditions/inputs for subsequent phases. The definition of the functional architecture of the intervention is then matched by a time plan, to be defined, of course, in a way that is consistent with the scanning and interconnection between the different operations involved in the intervention. Obviously, the more complex interventions are, the more it is generally appropriate to specify and agree on their logical-functional architecture. However, the timing and functional architecture of the intervention are no less relevant aspects in the case of interventions aimed at individuals. To limit ourselves to a paradigmatic case, psychotherapy lends itself to being thought of according to a series of phases. For example, the clinician may find it useful to focus initially on the critical situation that motivated the request as a preliminary and propaedeutic condition of a subsequent process of analysis and elaboration of the overall mode of relating to the client's world. An important aspect related to the dimension of time is the management of its chronological component, i.e., the schedule of events – who, and according to what criteria, establishes the temporal placement of operations, the decision about their possible displacement or cancellation. In this regard, the current authors have developed the conviction of the usefulness of agreeing upstream with the client system not only the schedule of activities but also the procedure by which to manage changes in the calendar of activities; this was a result of several circumstances in which the failure to carry out a planned event (for example, a meeting) resulted in the difficulty of restoring the flow of planned activities.

Third, like any organization, the intervention requires a *system of governance* – that is, a device/structure to make decisions necessary to manage the contingent aspects of the intervention. Every intervention takes place within changing situations, and therefore several of its aspects may need to be adapted to changing circumstances. Being clear about who has responsibility for such decisions and by what procedure they should be made is a factor that, in many cases, plays a significant role in the success of the intervention. Accordingly, in interventions involving a plurality of actors and stakeholders, it can be useful to foresee the building of a committee to preside over the monitoring of activities and decisions regarding their adaptation to changing contextual conditions.

Fourth, the organization comprising the intervention is characterized by a pattern, more or less explicit, of *processes* of *horizontal integration*, i.e., procedures and devices designed to promote, preserve, and consolidate coordination among the parallel operations that contribute to the pursuit of goals. Consider, for example, an intervention motivated by an adolescent's situation of distress, spread over different plans of action, each carried out by one or more professionals – for example, individual work with the adolescent, counseling provided to parents, counseling provided to teachers at the school attended by the adolescent, involvement of the adolescent in a creative socialization workshop. It is obvious that without proper coordination, these different courses of action may not only be less effective but may even hinder each other. Coordination is as much about practical and logistical aspects – mundanely, but no less importantly, preventing the timetables of the different actions from conflicting with each other – as it is about methodological aspects, that is, making sure that the different lines of action all move in the same direction.

Reporting

A hotly debated topic in the literature (e.g., Freda et al., 2013; Freda & Oberti, 2007; Grassi, 2004; Montesarchio & Venuleo, 2010; Salvatore, 2016a), reporting is considered the necessary complement of the psychologist's professional action (Carli, 2007).

One understands the expression "necessary complement" if one sees the intervention as a product of social exchange and, therefore, of a dynamic of sensemaking. If one moves away from the positivist-empiricist idea of the objectivity of the observation (for a criticism of this standpoint, see Gergen, 1985) and assumes that upstream of observation is the observer's point of view – namely, the dynamics of sensemaking in which the action of the person making the observation is embedded – one grasps the need to devote time to reconstructing the psychologist' interpretation of the action performed. The intervention is an action that – as happens with any service (Norman, 1986) – is marked by the simultaneity between production and consumption, thus by the lack of a period in which to verify the product supplied before its use. Add to this the fact that psychological intervention, as a professional action, is based on the agreement of the scientific community (Giannone & Lo Verso, 1998) and, therefore, on the necessity to make what has been accomplished visible.

We can, therefore, define the reporting of the intervention as *the representation of the professional action through the specification of the criteria guiding it.* The objects of the reporting cover the request received and its reformulation into a psychological problem that the psychologist considers suitable to address, the service provided designed by the psychologist, the processes implemented to this end, and the results achieved, all making explicit the interrelationship with the client that mediates the professional action.

Given these premises, reporting may take many forms, depending on the recipient and the objective being pursued. In this regard, the literature proposes numerous distinctions, which we summarize by differentiating situations where one accounts for one's work within the professional community of psychologists from situations where one gives an account of one's intervention to subjects related to other contexts of action and interest. The representation of the recipient of the report serves as a model for the writer since it anticipates the possible construction of meaning that the addressee will give to the text (Eco, 1975). In other words, reporting within one's professional community (for training, supervision, scientific writing) allows one to adopt a certain type of language not necessarily appropriate and understandable to other interlocutors (e.g., reporting aimed at a funder commissioning the intervention is quite different from one that is written to be read by a judge).

The reader model, together with the objective pursued, also guides the choice of the report's subject (e.g., the way funds were spent, use of resources, critical event, first interview, etc.) and the choice of the most appropriate spatial/temporal scale. On the latter point, think of a continuum where, at one end, there is the use of a magnifying glass to focus intensely on the details of short sequences of actions, and at the other, the use of a drone which one details backgrounds and brings to the fore the global process and its evolution.

Finally, the report can take different narrative styles chosen according to the conditions previously described. For instance, a historical approach may be preferred when linked to significant events or aimed at highlighting individual stages; alternatively, when the intervention is multi-faced, the report can be designed on a grid architecture rather than in a linear fashion to distinguish evolutive trajectories showing the different lines of action.

The validation of the intervention

We could summarize what has been expressed in the preceding paragraphs by stating that an intervention is the expression of a project (conceptual and organizational) that fits into a network of relationships (those related to the professional's organization and those of the client system) with the ambition of achieving a goal. By speaking of ambition, we recognize that the realization of the intervention corresponds to what was envisaged in the project only rarely (Grasso et al., 2016). This is due to the fact that the intervention unfolds through the mediation of an intersubjective field, which shapes the meanings and, therefore, the ways of feeling, thinking, and acting of the actors involved.

Therefore, it seems to us that intervention validation can be recognized as a necessity on the part of every professional. Its function is both to provide feedback on one's own work and to contribute to the empowerment/revisitation of the theoretical and methodological framework adopted.

For greater clarity and taking up what we have proposed elsewhere (Grasso et al., 2016), in what follows we will try to pinpoint the different elements (who, when, how, why, what), which, taken together, constitute the validation of the intervention, distinguishing between verification and evaluation.

In this direction, we designate as *verification* the analysis of the output generated by the intervention. Verification can be carried out at the conclusion of the intervention but also during the monitoring (process analysis) that accompanies it.

We define *evaluation* as the judgment regarding the impact of usefulness/appropriateness/soundness attributed to the intervention by the client system and/or the system the professional refers to (on the distinction between outcome and impact, see Chapter 5). It is worth noting that the client/professional system may consist of numerous figures (client, funder, stakeholders, etc.), each of which represents a specific point of view (see Chapter 5). Consider, for example, the cost/benefit ratio and the value it may have for the different actors involved (e.g., client/insurer). Accordingly, it seems useful to emphasize that evaluation should not be understood as a datum, descriptive of what happened, but as a situated action, expressing the position of the actor towards the intervention provided (Salvatore & Scotto Di Carlo, 2005).

In short, as we have already mentioned, verification, evaluation, and their interconnection can be useful in looking at one's work with a critical gaze. In this direction, critical events, which do not seem to have worked as we expected, as well as what worked beyond our expectations, become the most useful clues to empower our model of intervention.

3 The idiographic and abductive character of the intervention

As noted in Chapter 1, the prevailing tendency in contemporary psychology is to view the relationship between scientific knowledge and intervention in applicative terms, i.e., to conceive of professional action as aimed at using knowledge already available, produced in the context of research. In many circumstances, the applicative logic is functional to the goals and conditions of intervention. For example, the Italian Psychological Association's paper critiquing anti-migration policies referred to previously (Section 1) is an example of the practical application of knowledge made available by research. In many other cases, however, the intervention builds on and is conducted because of contingent issues and local and situated events, which are, by definition, unique in their idiosyncratic specificity. In these cases, the application logic shows its limitation in a way that is all the more relevant, the greater the effort required to adapt the contingent to the Procrustean bed of predefined knowledge (which by definition concerns general classes of phenomena). In such cases, the understanding of the problem to be addressed, due to the specificity of its local form as well as of the project conducted on it by the actors involved, is a constitutive part of the professional action. Accordingly, *the intervention takes on the character of a social process of knowledge construction.*

If this is so, what is the mode that organizes such a process of knowledge construction?

Our answer is that *knowledge for and in the intervention is idiographic in nature, grounded on abduction* (Salvatore, 2016b). We discuss this idea in what follows with reference to the thesis that, with others, one of us has developed about the need to overcome the idiographic-nomothetic dichotomy through the enhancement of abductive logic (e.g., Salvatore & Valsiner, 2009, 2010).

Idiographic and nomothetic. A misleading juxtaposition

Historically, the idiographic approach has been associated with the recognition of the uniqueness of the subject of inquiry: if nomothetic knowledge is about regularities detected in terms of general laws, idiographic knowledge is understanding of the particular, of the individual event, and of what happened, taken in its uniqueness.

> [T]he empirical sciences seek in the knowledge of reality either the general in the form of natural law or the particular in the historically determined

form. They consider in one part the ever-enduring form, in the other part the unique content, determined within itself, of an actual happening. The one comprises sciences of law, the other sciences of events; the former teaches what always is, the latter what once was. If one may resort to neologisms, it can be said that scientific thought is in one case nomothetic, in the other idiographic.

(Windelband, 1904/1998, p. 13)

Subsequently, the notion of uniqueness has been interpreted as opposed to generalization, as if idiographic knowledge is not knowledge of the *unique* but is *unique*, that is, knowledge that does not involve any form of generalization (Salvatore & Valsiner, 2009, 2010). However, this interpretation, which implicitly overlaps uniqueness and singularity, is problematic. It, in fact, does not consider that any instance of knowledge is inherently a form of generalization. It also fails to consider that the very fact of recognizing an event requires linking it to a class: to say that something is unique implies the use of a criterion. Each individual event is recognized as unique through the conceptual linkages of similarity and difference it has with other objects. For example, representing the Battle of Waterloo – and treating it as a unique event – implies treating it as a battle, i.e., identifying a trait of equivalence and, at the same time, a trait of difference from other events (the many battles that have occurred in human history) (for a critical discussion of the opposition between idiographic and nomothetic, focusing on the use of the notion in the context of clinical psychology, see Thornton, 2008).

The interpretation of uniqueness, as opposed to generalization, must be contextualized to the state of scientific debate in the early 20th century. The contemporary scientific context requires a different reading, one that avoids the *cul-de-sac* to which the confusion between unique and singular leads. In this perspective, it is useful to refer to the idea of processes as emerging from fundamental dynamics because of field conditions (see Chapter 1). This idea leads to the interpretation of the notion of uniqueness in terms of *contingency*. Accordingly, a phenomenon is unique not because it is the exemplar of a class of N=1 cardinality; rather, it is unique in the sense that its occurrence is the event happening in a given spatial-temporal surround, which realizes the fundamental dynamics within and because of local conditions. Since field conditions are never the same, constantly changing with the irreversible course of time, no event can ever be the same as another event. This means that the interpretation we propose of uniqueness in terms of contingency does not deny the singularity of the event. However, it broadens the point of view, shifting the focus from the empirical content of the event to the field dynamics from which it emerges. In short, the focus shifts from asking: in what terms and to what extent is this empirical event (dis)similar to other events? to ask: *from what field dynamic does this event emerge, and what is it an expression of?*

Take, for example, an event of conflict within an organization. According to the approach proposed here, it is not a matter of identifying the general category of similar episodes to which to assimilate the event to apply the knowledge related to the category to the event; rather, it is a matter of analyzing the local form (i.e., what we have called *process*, see Chapter 1) that the dynamics of sensemaking has acquired within that specific field of human activity (the life of the organization). In other words, it is a matter of modeling *that* event in terms of the contingent emergence of the fundamental dynamics.

Modelling the link between dynamics and event

The interpretation of the notion of uniqueness in terms of contingency has an important theoretical implication, partly highlighted in Chapter 1. Contingent events that instantiate the fundamental dynamics do not resemble each other in terms of their empirical content. They can also be radically different because of the different field conditions that preside over their emergence. This means that we regard them as belonging to the same general class not because of their empirical similarity but because of the possibility of modeling them as forms emerging from the same fundamental dynamics. Just as the movement of the planets around the sun and falling off the scooter are entirely dissimilar empirically and yet conceptualizable as exemplars of the same general class (they are contingent instantiations of gravity), in the same way, populism and petting one's dog are events that are as incommensurable on the empirical level as they are assimilable to the class of instantiations of the dynamics of sensemaking. In short, the link between events and dynamics is modeling, rather than empirical – intensional, rather than extensional (Salvatore, 2016c). This means that dynamics cannot be regarded as the generalized prototype of events that can be associated with it, defined by means of the collection of a plurality of elements (where the accumulation of exemplars serves to marginalize their differences). Rather, dynamics should be considered a superordinate interpretive model: the general semantics by which the local event becomes modellable. In sum, unlike the empirical (extensional) criterion, according to which the general class is defined by the empirical quality shared by the exemplars, the modeling (intentional) criterion qualifies the general class because exemplars can be interpreted in terms of the model.

The shift from the empirical to the modeling criterion has an important methodological consequence for intervention – more generally, for the production of scientific knowledge in the field of psychology. The analysis of the dynamics cannot be based on empirical regularities across cases. Instead, it is necessary to analyze the cases in a situated way, namely by reason of the local conditions under which they occur. At the same time, this kind of situated analysis needs to be performed framed in the general semantics offered by the general model of the dynamics. This brings to the forefront the way abductive logic operates and its integrative role between idiographic and nomothetic (Salvatore & Valsiner, 2010).

Abduction and intervention

According to the thesis we are discussing here, idiographic knowledge is not a form of knowledge construction that rejects generalization (which would be an oxymoron, as noted previously). Rather, it is a form of knowledge construction that uses abduction to generalize through contingency.

Abduction is a type of inference that reconstructs the event/phenomenon based on available empirical clues. Abductive inference goes back from effects to causes – it aims to reconstruct the occurrence of a particular cause (present or past), the presence of which makes the available clues significant.

> It must be remembered that abduction, although it is very little hampered by logical rules, nevertheless is logical inference, asserting its conclusion only problematically or conjecturally. It is true, but nevertheless having a perfectly definite logical form.
> . . . The form of inference, therefore, is this:
> The surprising fact, C, is observed;
> But if A were true, C would be a matter of course,
>
> Hence, there is reason to suspect that A is true.
> *(Peirce, 1902/1932a, CP 5.188–189)*

In other words, the reconstruction of the cause is done by assuming that its occurrence makes the co-occurrence of the clues meaningful. Consider the investigator who observed pieces of glass on the floor, a broken windowpane, and footprints spread around the room. These co-occurring clues are in themselves dumb, meaningless, part of the same background in which infinite other elements (e.g., the color of the walls, the temperature of the room) coexist. As the investigator conjectures, circumstance A – "the murderer entered through the window, breaking the glass" – is capable of tying the clues together in a plausible gestalt – what Peirce (1897/1932a) calls the *unification of predicates* – these clues acquire meaning and, consequently, the circumstance A takes on the value of an (possible) explanation of what happened.

It is worth highlighting how abductive and inductive inference differs and how they are similar. Inductive inference treats empirical elements with the aim of extracting from them what they have in common, the local regularity, which is, in turn, used to infer the general law. Peirce (1897/1932a) defines this inference operation as *habit formation*. Unlike inductive inference, abductive inference is not aimed at producing the general law. Rather, it uses the general law (i.e., the model of the dynamics) to interpret the clues in order to produce a pattern of the local event that occurred: the local model of the contingent event. In summary, both induction and abduction start from empirical data. Induction uses such data to arrive at the general law as a generalization of the local rule (the local rule consists of the similarity between the empirical elements collected); abduction approaches the empirical data to construct the local model of the process that generated it, using the semantics offered by the general theory for this purpose.

Abductive inference starts, therefore, from the same point as inductive inference: the empirical data. However, it follows a different path to arrive at a different form of knowledge. Abduction aims to produce the local model – that is, an understanding of the process that determines the event – it does not use the event to arrive at the general rule; rather, it uses the general rule to understand the event (Eco, 1975). Abductive inference does this through three operations (Salvatore, 2014):

- the pertinentization of salient occurrences;
- the gestaltic connection of salient occurrences;
- the reconstructive interpretation of them in terms of the dynamics from which they presumably emerge.

The three operations are closely intertwined, or rather, they are components of the same epistemic process – each is accomplished through the others. To return to the investigator's example, it can be seen that the identification of clues (pertinentization) and their gestaltic interconnection, as components of the same past event (reconstruction), are sides of the same dice.

This highlights the specificity of generalization by abduction: the interpretation of the clues in terms of reconstruction of the inferred phenomenon (unification of predicates, in Peirce's terms) is a form of abstraction, that is, the operation of making only certain aspects/properties of the clues relevant, those that serve for modeling and reconstruction (for the definition of abstraction in terms of relevance, see Bühler, 1934/1990). For example, the investigator in the previous example abstracts from the pieces of glass only one of the infinite qualities that could be attributed to them: the property of their coming from the window.

It is important to take into account that abductive abstraction requires a general law in order to be implemented – it is, in fact, the general law that guides the selection of properties to be made pertinent. This leads to the conclusion that abduction can be conceived as a form of *generalizing abstraction*: cases are abstracted to acquire the form/status of local and contingent exemplification of the general law. This is the sense of considering abduction a form of modeling generalization: the general class that collects the cases is not defined in terms of the empirical similarity among cases (as happens in induction) but of a conceptual principle (the general rule).

Intervention as abduction

The previous discussion allows us to enrich the meaning of the distinction between dynamics and phenomenon presented in Chapter 1 (Section 2). The theory of sensemaking (see Chapters 2 and 3) provides the general law describing the universal and invariant mode of operation of the dynamics proposed as the object of psychological science. The psychologist grappling with a client refers to the general rule in order to have an interpretive framework by means of which to understand the contingency of the client's local world abductively. Such understanding is proposed as an innovative glimpse into the client's world, conveying semiotic innovation, potentially capable of nurturing developmental perspectives.

This leads to the conclusion that psychological intervention, where it is configured as a social practice of knowledge construction, can be considered an *act of abduction*. This is in three complementary senses.

First, abduction is the way professional action functions. The design and mode of how professional action is exercised – for example, the interpretation of the demand, the setting of the goal, the manner in which the client relationship is organized – is based on the interpretation of the client's world. As seen previously, this interpretation can be made in two different ways: inductively or abductively. In the first way, the client's world is treated as an exemplar of a general psychological category (e.g., a nosography class, a behavioral category, the class defined by a certain score range on a given test) and the characteristics associated with the category are projected onto the case. In short, the case becomes the application of universal knowledge. When abductive interpretation is involved, the case is understood as a contingent event: psychological knowledge is used to reconstruct the idiosyncratic and local process through which elements of the client's experience (along with others that in this way become representable) acquire meaning, both synchronic and diachronic.

Second, abduction is the outcome of the intervention. The professional psychological function ultimately aims to promote in the client an innovative gaze with which they can view the world in further ways. As is obvious, semiotic innovation cannot be accomplished by transmitting ready-made packages of specialized knowledge. Semiotic innovation is not a single outcome but a process – it returns in this regard to what was pointed out by Carli (1987b), who defined the goal of psychological intervention as *methodological*: the development of a way of thinking about experience. This means that the crux of psychological intervention is not the content of the interpretation to which the client arrives, but the development of their competence to interpret experience in its contingency – in short, the development of their competence to make abduction.

Third, abduction is how professional practice functions as a lever in the development of general psychological theory. General psychological theory is not a model defined once-and-for-all. It evolves according to a multiplicity of developmental paths, each conceivable as a form of generalization – for example, the relationships that the model detects can be better specified and differentiated; its scope of validity can be limited or expanded; relationships of equivalence and/or complementarity can be established with other models, and so on. However, abduction does not directly aim at the construction of general models. This does not mean that it renounces generalization. Rather, the development of the general theory is the side product, so to speak, of the systematic activity of building local models. This point has been discussed by one of us in previous papers (Salvatore & Valsiner, 2009, 2010). We will, therefore, confine ourselves here to briefly recalling the terms of the issue. Every contingent event to be modeled is a challenge posed to the general theory and to its ability to frame its interpretation. Thus, the development of the general theory is fueled by the fact that it is systematically called upon to work at the service of constructing knowledge of the contingent. In other words, the development of the general theory is motivated, channeled, and validated by the terms of the epistemic demand placed on it to provide semantics and syntax useful for generating the local model of contingent phenomena. Historically, until the end of World War II (Toomela, 2007), psychological science largely functioned in this way, as shown by the work of giants such as Freud, Piaget, Vygotsky, and Werner. Our idea is that psychological intervention can offer an opportunity to recover what is innovative and creative in such a logic – the professional action as a source of endless opportunities for the development of the general theory, challenged in its ability to ground the effort to expand the client's semiotic resources.

5
THEORY OF THE CLIENT

This chapter is devoted to the theory of the client, the part of GTPI that models the relationship between the psychologist and the actors involved in the intervention. Central to the theory of the client is the recognition of the distance that exists between the commonsensical theories that motivate and shape the demand that actors – individuals, organizations, and institutions – address to psychology and the interpretive models and methods of intervention with which the latter responds to that demand. As we shall have occasion to point out, this distance varies; however, in many circumstances, it manifests itself in terms of an epistemic conflict between viewpoints that tend to be incommensurable with each other – common sense versus scientific knowledge. Hence, there is a need to conceptualize the relationship between client and psychologist and the specificity that this relationship assumes within psychological intervention. Modeling the concepts of client and request in psychological terms fulfills this purpose. On this basis, it becomes possible, on the one hand, to analyze how the client and psychologist's projects can interact in order to generate value and, on the other hand, how to promote the development of the client as a function of the intervention's requirements for effectiveness and usefulness.

The chapter is divided into six parts. The first section introduces the topic of the client's request and highlights its specificity in the field of psychology. The second section proposes the conceptualization of the constructs of *demand* at the core of the psychological model of the client's request. In the third section, the theme of the value of the intervention as a function of the relationship between client and intervention is explored. The fourth and fifth sections propose a view of the development of the client's request and some methodological criteria that can be used for this purpose. The sixth section

DOI: 10.4324/9781003449362-6

completes the discussion of the client's development by illustrating the role that the analysis of the demand plays in this perspective.

1 The client's request

The request is an aspect that concerns any profession and, more generally, any activity of providing goods and services – such activities exist to the extent that someone requests them or otherwise expresses willingness/interest in enjoying them. In the case of psychological intervention, however, requesting professional service has peculiar characteristics, which deserve to be understood and given due consideration in professional action.

The normative weakness of the psychology profession

We owe Carr-Saunders (1928) for the idea that professionals are distinguished from other workers and intellectuals by reason of a "specialized skill" based on scientific knowledge. Similarly, Greenwood (1957) highlights five attributes typical of professions: the actions of a professional are 1) based on a specific body of theoretical-practical knowledge; 2) acquired as part of a higher education path that allows them to have authority over the client; 3) garner recognition by the community; 4) authority and recognition are regulated by a code of ethics; and 5) by the establishment of agencies that build the institutional and cultural infrastructure of the profession. On this basis, Western countries have constructed a model of work that is clearly distinct from that envisioned by Taylorism, built around the figure of the practitioner and the lawyer, which enabled the recognition and protection of the professions in the industrial period (1945–1975) (Piketty, 2013/2014).

Over the years, multiple authors have tried to redefine the concept of the profession, considering the different professions, the variable working conditions, the reinterpretations made by the agencies in relation to which the professional functions are practiced, and the market conditions regulating them (Bellini & Maestripieri, 2018). While there have been questions about their function in societies, the professions have also been analyzed by emphasizing their pursuit of status and privileges. However, it is interesting to note that what remains, in the different definitions, is the presence of specialized knowledge, acquired through a course of study, that enables the professional to produce normative statements in different areas – from birth to conflict, from physical and mental health to recreation, and from education to peacekeeping, just to give a few examples (Evetts, 2003).

The specialized knowledge that distinguishes the professional from the layperson implies that any professional action involves a degree of epistemic conflict between client and professional – i.e., an inherent divergence about how to interpret the problem motivating the request, the function, forms, and manner of professional action. If this were not the case, clients would have no reason to appeal to the professional: they would be able to deal with the issue on their own.

In the case of most professions, however, epistemic conflict is regulated effectively by established cultural and institutional devices whose normativity frames the exchange between client and expert. Two such fundamental devices are the *socio-symbolic* and *institutional status* enjoyed by professional systems – the power that such status fosters – and the *simplified incorporation within common sense of elements of the scientific knowledge the profession is based on* – what social representations theory regards as the product of the joint processes of anchoring and objectification (Moscovici, 1961/1976).

The combined operation of these two devices means that the client generally acknowledges the professional's epistemic and socio-institutional power, recognizing her/him as the one who has the final word about the interpretation of the problem, the way and timing of dealing with it, and the regulation of the relationship (e.g., management of time and space, fee, mode of communication). If the engineer approached by a client has reached the conclusion that, for reasons of statics, the wall cannot be torn down, the client may well try to insist but will eventually recognize that assessment as a fact (also if they decide not to follow it, they consider their decision a deviation from the rule). This is because, on the one hand, the client recognizes the professional's authority derived from possessing the scientific knowledge necessary for the assessment, and, on the other hand, they nonetheless have a naïve theory of the problem, which makes the expert's scientific knowledge and its value representable – the client may not know Newton's law and the theory of general relativity but is fully aware that, if not properly supported, objects have the bad habit of not remaining suspended in the air. Such practical knowledge is not enough to ground an expert decision, but it is sufficient to make the client recognize that an expert decision is needed and to give it normative value.

We can thus come to the following conclusion – the actions of many professionals may take the client and their request for granted; they need not concern themselves with the management of the relationship with it since that function is accomplished as if automatically, operated by default by the institutional and cultural system in which both professional and client are embedded. Incidentally, several critical issues that professional systems face today can be interpreted as consequences of the progressive weakening of the instituted status that society attributes to them, thus of the emergence of the client as a conflictual element that needs to be regulated by and from within the professional action (for an analysis of the institutional dynamic of the practitioner-patient relationship and its crisis, see Venezia et al., 2019; for a similar analysis related to the role of the teacher, see Salvatore & Scotto di Carlo, 2005).

Psychological intervention is also in a position, under certain circumstances, to anchor itself in the symbolic regulation devices proper to "strong" professions. An emblematic example in this sense comes from psychotherapy, whose assimilation to the medical role offers a powerful normative and epistemic anchorage with which to regulate the relationship with the client. Those who turn to the psychotherapist do so because of a theory about their condition, as well as about the way they relate to the professional, the behavior expected of them, the value of their work, codified in common sense and conveyed by social representations that, although subject to some deterioration (Venezia et al., 2019), are still powerfully shared in society. In short, in the context of psychotherapy, the psychologist does not need to organize the client's request (except in marginal respects) – common sense takes care of that: the client already comes to psychotherapy as a patient because they possess, in their cultural repertoire, the practical knowledge foundational to that form of request. In other circumstances, the psychologist's regulative power in the request is institutional in nature. These are the cases in which the psychologist operates at the behest of agencies that exercise regulatory functions towards recipients of interventions – for example, consider the psychological work in the justice system or, again, the activity of psychologists called upon to certify the prerequisites necessary to access certain types of health treatment (e.g., bariatric surgery).

However, taken as a whole, it should be recognized that the psychological profession does not have the same access to client regulation devices that other professional systems enjoy. The psychological profession has a weaker socio-symbolic and institutional status (Salvatore, 2006). This is not the place to dwell on the historical and structural causes of such a weak social status. We will simply point out that the professional psychological action is not easily representable in its specificity, both because the operations that the psychologist performs are in most cases assimilated by common sense to scripts typical of everyday life – for example, think of clients who represent their conversation with the psychologist as a chat with a friend or dialogue with the confessor – and because it is difficult, if not impossible, to identify a clear connection between what the psychologist does and what the client gets out of that doing. If the medical practitioner recommends an antibiotic and, after a few days, the patient no longer has flu symptoms, the means-result connection is easy to grasp. Rarely is such a connection possible in relation to the psychologist's actions. Moreover, it must be acknowledged that psychology and psychologists make their own contribution to the institutional weakness of the profession by fuelling, rather than counteracting, the fragmentation of disciplinary language and scientific knowledge (see Chapter 1).

Due to the relative socio-institutional weakness of psychology, the requests addressing it do not find adequate channeling, either on the representational level (what anticipatory image the client expresses towards the psychologist), the normative level (what the client considers legitimate to ask of the psychologist) or the pragmatic level (what mode of regulation of the relationship the client proposes to the psychologist). As a result, in many cases, the requests that reach the psychologist prove to have traits of incompatibility or at least conflicting elements with respect to the possibility of designing appropriate professional actions on the proposed problems. It is not unusual for people to turn to the psychologist with unrealistic goals, with the expectation that the psychologist can (and is willing) to manipulate third parties (children, employees, clients); it is not uncommon for a person to turn to the psychologist with instrumental and demonstrative purposes; in organizational and institutional contexts, the request for psychological intervention is part of and conveys the inevitably conflicting dynamic between the points of view involved (e.g., between management and staff, between commercial and technical areas). During a supervisory meeting, a colleague working in a family counseling center recounted that he had received a request from the judge for an expert opinion, phrased in a question of this kind: "The moral rectitude of the woman should be assessed, for the purpose of verifying her suitability for the parental role."

In our view, in such circumstances, the psychologist needs to mobilize a function of elaboration of the client's request in order to optimize its compatibility with the minimal conditions the intervention needs if it is to generate value.

The (bearable) lightness of psychology

In many cases, the psychologist's intervention is kept within areas of compatibility with common sense. Return in this regard to the traffic accident prevention intervention described in Chapter 3 – the goal of the intervention is to change the tendency of motorcyclists to drive at high speeds by working on their attitudes and social norms through awareness campaigns and enhancing the opinion of influential personalities. Now, in that case, both the explanation of the phenomenon and, even more so, the solutions put forward are fully consistent with common sense. They have been formulated on the basis of empirical analysis, but without requiring a major shift from naïve theory about how people function – naïve theory, let us remark, each of us possesses not because we are psychologists but because we have assimilated the practical knowledge available in the cultural milieu in which we grew up. For example, the prediction that the message of an influential personality can change the attitudes/standpoints of bikers may prove right (though we must be allowed some skepticism), but nevertheless, it remains a belief that one need not have studied psychology to hold.

Keeping the epistemic conflict subthreshold – i.e., responding to clients with interpretive models and methods immediately consistent with client expectations – is the way in which psychology professionals do not infrequently find it necessary to operate, given the profession's weak institutional conditions. More generally, however, it is a strategy that offers the advantage of reducing the social distance between the client and the psychologist. Underlying it is the idea that if the psychologist and the client share the same premises of sense, this will lead both of them to take their relationship for granted. Obviously, this relationship will still require adjustment; however, the adjustment will concern only marginal aspects, the variability of which will remain within the margins of the shared premises of sense. Ultimately, then, a subthreshold of epistemic conflict allows the client to represent their own expectation mirrored by the psychologist's response and for the latter to treat the client as a given condition, grounding the psychologist's actions (rather than a goal to be pursued). Consider in this sense the multiple appearances of psychologists in the media. Often, what is expected from them is that they legitimize commonsensical interpretations through their reformulation in vaguely technical-scientific language.

All this can be understood if one considers that in the case of psychological intervention, the epistemic conflict has traits of potential radicality. The practical knowledge that fuels the request for psychology has a foundational value of identity and social regulation: the beliefs that (individual and collective) subjects have about phenomena of psychological interest are at the core of the way they make sense of themselves and the world. Consider the essential role that the development of the theory of mind plays in ontogeny; again, consider how the knowledge we have of how the mind works is integral to the metacognitive functions that organize cognitive processes (Cornoldi, 1995). Ultimately, what we believe our mind is and how it works is the substance of what each of us feels to be the foundation of how we understand and relate to what happens in interpersonal relationships, at work, and in society. It can, therefore, be well understood that in circumstances where scientific knowledge about psychological phenomena comes into epistemic conflict with common sense, this conflict can be a potential source of profound destabilization, which impacts the premises of sense operating as the foundation of subjectivity. We have learned that elementary particles interact at a distance, that bodies of different weights have the same falling speed, that weighing oneself on the Moon and weighing oneself on Earth do not produce the same result, that organisms are made largely of water, and that an increase of a few degrees in the average temperature of the globe generates catastrophic eco-systemic effects. These and many other pieces of counterintuitive knowledge challenge our naïve theories concerning natural events. However, learning them does not turn our sense of ourselves upside-down (unless we are researchers who, as a result of such learnings, are forced to abandon theories to whose development we have devoted our lives) since none of them is constitutive of the way we see ourselves. Consider, by contrast, psychological knowledge – to limit ourselves to a few concepts of those recalled in the preceding pages of this book: the idea that our thoughts are not produced inside our heads but are a function of the intersubjective field, the idea that meaning is not prior to its expression but emerges from what we say and do, the idea that contents of experience do not reflect an objective world but are the product of a continuous and recursive process of pertinentization. Concepts of this kind do not have a marginal impact on our identity – taking them seriously, they profoundly deconstruct the experience we have of ourselves. They place us in the same condition of radical subversion of experience suffered by Thomas Anderson (Neo) when Morpheus reveals the reality of the Matrix to him.

The pressure to conform to common sense that psychological intervention undergoes can thus be interpreted as mirroring the radically innovative impact that the psychological gaze on human affairs is potentially capable of expressing. There are reasons, however, to argue that it is preferable for psychological intervention to follow Neo's choice and opt for the red pill, the one that marks the decision to push beyond the Herculean columns of the socio-culturally instituted view of things. Beyond the metaphor, the psychological intervention has not only the need but also, above all, the interest in conceiving of the client's request – the epistemic conflict that substantiates the relationship with it – as a process to be elaborated and promoted in a word: governed, rather than an exogenous event to be neutralized and/or taken for granted. This is for two complementary reasons.

On the one hand, as much applies to psychology as to the professions in general. The magnitude of the epistemic conflict with the client's request plays a relevant role in determining the value of the professional function: the more the epistemic distance between the professional knowledge and the commonsensical practical knowledge, the more the former acquires value, insofar as it cannot be surrogated by common sense. Those who have not trained for this purpose are unable to fly a plane, play the piano, design a building, diagnose a disease, or calculate the trajectory of an asteroid; they must consequently turn to those who possess such skills. From this point of view, one of the causes and, at the same time, of the symptoms of the weak socio-institutional value of the psychological profession is the tendency, widespread in society, to consider psychological knowledge as part of everyone's experiential repertoire. How many times have we heard "being a bit of a psychologist" evoked as one of the skills that qualify the most disparate of occupations – from soccer coach to entrepreneur, from teacher to policeman, from taxi driver to merchant?

On the other hand, in a variety of circumstances, the request is simply not there or is otherwise weak. In the collective imagination, and thus in the representations of potential clients, many issues and problems on which psychology could make a relevant contribution are preferentially associated with other scientific-professional fields. Think of, to limit ourselves to a few examples, issues related to occupational safety, the design and management of organizational processes, urban planning, the relationship between citizens and institutions, and the territorial governance of environmental resources – topics that are thought to be predominantly the responsibility of engineers, biochemists, lawyers, political scientists, etc. A few years ago, one of us, in the context of a project to experiment with the psychological function in schools, had the opportunity to meet with several school principals to agree on possible psychological interventions at the schools they directed (Salvatore, 2001). Invariably, the principals would arrive at such meetings with the idea that the psychologist's role was to take charge of individual students' behavioral problems. The interaction with these principals allowed us, in most cases, to elaborate on this initial expectation and to agree on a plurality of psychological interventions in relation to problems concerning the empowerment of the teaching-learning settings, the governance of organizational dynamics, and the relationship with families and the territory. As one of the school heads commented, "I had no idea that psychologists dealt with these issues!" Today, thanks in part to projects of that kind, many school principals have a broader idea of the psychological function.

The opportunity to promote the request of psychological intervention in areas not traditionally associated with psychological expertise is made even more cogent by the profound socio-institutional transformations taking place in contemporary societies, which have led to the emergence of critical phenomena and instances of development that need to be understood and governed. Think of strategic issues such as the aging of the population, global demographic growth, the redefinition of socioeconomic development models in terms of sustainability, the demographic, sociocultural, and economic impact of migration flows, and the new perspectives drawn by robotics and artificial intelligence. On such issues, it is the system of psychology as a whole that has the opportunity – and we would add, the political and ethical duty (Di Maria, 2021) – to provide a contribution. This requires, on the one hand, the development of an innovative interpretative framework and intervention models and, on the other, the ability to promote social interest and investment in them. From this point of view, the institutional weakness of psychology can become a strategic advantage in the ability to move flexibly and innovatively across the developmental trajectories outlined by contemporary upheavals. Lightness, then, as a condition and as a method – what is needed to project oneself into the future with something to tell and at the same time without "losing unity," as the filmmaker Antonio Capuano enjoins the young aspiring colleague Fabio (Sorrentino, 2021).

2 Request and demand

In the previous section, we discussed reasons why it is appropriate for psychological intervention not to take the client's request for granted but to equip itself with a function to elaborate the request. However, the conception of the client's request as a process to be elaborated rather than taken for granted raises the question of how such governance can be achieved. GTPI considers this issue to be internal to its own domain of interest; that is to say, the elaboration of the client's request for psychological intervention, however much it may take advantage of methods and tools developed in other scientific fields, nevertheless deserves to be modeled from a psychological standpoint. We devote the remainder of this section to presenting a model to be used to this end.

Request and demand from a psychological perspective

The GTPI model of the client's request can be summed up by the following tenets.

First, the client's request does not concern only the content of what the client asks of the psychologist. The GTPI sees the request as denoting the whole relationship with the psychologist that the client proposes to the professional by asking something as it unfolds over the whole space-time arc of the intervention. The request, therefore, implies the socio-organizational, pragmatic, and economic facets that sustain and substantiate the way the client addresses the psychological function and psychologists; the type and extent of resources (time, money, reputation) that the client invests in the intervention, their behavior, the formal and informal norms they expect to be adopted, the evaluations they express, the modes they regulate the relation with the psychologist, etc. Understood in this way, the concept of request helps to recognize the two-dimensional nature of the intervention. On the one hand, the intervention has an *operative* component – that is, the productive action of the professional aimed at pursuing the purpose. In Chapter 4, we proposed a typology of the content of such actions, grouped into three levels of semiotic change. On the other hand, the intervention involves an *organizational* component aimed at governing the relationship with the client and its request over time. As is obvious, the two components are not separate pieces of reality; rather, they are constructs to be used for modeling how the exchange between client and psychologist works and how to govern it according to the purposes of the intervention. It is in these terms that we discuss them in what follows.

Second, the psycho-semiotic approach adopted in this volume leads us to recognize that the request is a *performative sign* – that is, a meaning conveyed by an act. Like any sign, the formulation of a request to the psychologist is grounded in a system of meaning working as a *premise of sense*: an abstract and generalized meaning that motivates and shapes the action of turning to the psychologist and, at the same time, makes sense of it in the eyes of whomever performs it. Following Carli and Paniccia (Carli, 1987a, 1987b, 1997; Carli & Paniccia, 2003), we define *demand* as the premise of sense underlying the request.

Economic theory has developed a definition of the term *demand* – the volume of consumption asked for by the market. One of the most relevant contributions that Renzo Carli made to the theory of psychological intervention was to propose a definition of the term from the perspective of psychological language – more specifically, psychoanalytic language. According to this definition, the demand is *the affective symbolization that feeds – and at the same time finds expression in – the request that the client addresses to the psychologist* (e.g., Carli, 1987a, 1987b, 1997; Carli & Paniccia, 2003).

Carli's conceptualization of the demand developed within the frame provided by the dual conception of meaning (see Chapter 1). After all, it could not have been otherwise – the psychology (e.g., Johnson-Laird, 1983) and psychoanalysis (e.g., Fornari, 1979) of the years in which he developed the theory of the demand were firmly rooted in Saussurian structuralist theory. According to this conception, all behavior is a sign composed of the combination of two planes – the plane of expression (signifier) and the plane of content (the signified) (Eco, 1975; see Chapter 2). Consistently with this premise, the demand was conceived as the signifier that expresses and conveys the demand as its unconscious meaning (for a discussion of the theories of meaning underlying the psychoanalytic theory, see Salvatore & Zittoun, 2011).

The triadic theory of meaning underlying the psycho-semiotic approach adopted in this volume leads to a reinterpretation, or rather, a further articulation of the psychological concept of demand. Three elements deserve to be highlighted in this regard.

First, triadic theory makes it possible to highlight the performative nature of the demand. Like any other meaning, demand is not only a behavior produced by the premise of sense of which it is part; it is also the way in which that premise of sense is reproduced over time. In other words, the demand does not convey meaning: it *produces* it within and through the intersubjective field it sustains.

Second, in the light of the triadic theory of meaning, the demand is worth considering a form of *significance in absentia*. This implies a generalization of the concept: the demand can be grasped not only at the level of affective symbolization – i.e., at the level of highest abstraction of the affective self-other schemata (see Chapter 3) but also at the level of less abstract meanings – hyper-generalized signs, generalized signs, domain beliefs (see Chapter 3), insofar as the latter are analyzed in their function of premises of sense underlying the client's interpretation of their condition and, therefore, of the request. It will depend on the conditions and objectives of the intervention to choose the level of abstraction at which to anchor the significance in absentia grounding the request.

Finally, the triadic theory helps to focus on the inherently intersubjective nature of demand. As *significance in absentia*, it operates as the foundation of the intersubjective field through the process of compatibilization of the pertinent dimensions of the client-psychologist relationship – the process we have previously termed *Pentecost effect* (see Chapter 3). This means that the client's demand is nonetheless able to use the intervention as a referent that can sustain the intersubjective field necessary for its own reproduction. The psychologist is not given the opportunity to prevent this since, just as one cannot not communicate, one cannot not collude. In other words, one cannot evade the intersubjective field generated by the other's interpretive activity; as discussed in Chapter 3, the function of the intervention is to introduce perturbations into that intersubjective field, not to eliminate it.

The concept of demand outlined previously has a central implication to thinking in psychological terms about the elaboration of the client's request and, more generally, about the psychologist's actions. Indeed, the psychological theory of the demand enables us to recognize that the decision of a subject to turn to the psychologist is a phenomenon that can be understood beyond the functional level – namely, such a decision is not only the consequence of an objective condition of necessity that the client recognizes and translates into consequent action. On the contrary, every request, no matter how much it may at the same time find justification on the functional level, is always *a performative exercise of subjectivity*: an act of signification, that is to say, an event produced by the client's interpretive activity.

Ultimately, to say that the request is grounded in and nurtured by demand amounts to saying that the client's decision to search for the professional service of a psychologist is not a mirror of objective reality but a product of how the subject makes sense of their own condition, where this process of making sense is exerted by mobilizing, among other signs, also the performative sign of becoming a client of the psychologist. This means that the *demand is not synonymous with need*. The need is the state of absence of a resource necessary for the subject's reproduction. One needs air, food, water, and shelter. When one claims to need resources that serve contingent goals (i.e., not associated with states of need) – "I need money," "I need the car," "I need my wife to love me" – one is actually producing a sign that conveys the normative absolutization of the desire, through its assimilation to a condition of need – X is so essential to my life in the same way that air is essential to keep me alive.

As Renzo Carli used to say – *there is no psychologist because there are clients; there are clients because there is a psychologist.* Psychology is not a given reality with which one enters a relationship as a consequence of another given reality (the need that motivates the request); rather, it is an element that lets the individual, by entering into a relationship with it, shape their own interpretation of themselves and their world. From this point of view, the psychologist's client operates like Neil Buchanan (https://it.wikipedia.org/wiki/Neil_Buchanan), the TV performer who produces assemblages of the most varied materials (buckets, gloves, sticks, straw), which, viewed from above, take the form of meaningful objects. In Buchanan's compositions, each of the materials used had its own functional value; at the same time, a different perspective (the overall view from above) enables the clear emergence of a different network of relationships among the components, which overlooks (without denying) their functionality and makes a further, global meaning come to light. Considering the client's request is like looking at Neil Buchanan's works from above – placing in the background the functional meaning conveyed by the client's concern in order to recognize the global subjective meaning it conveys.

A map of the demand

Carli and his colleagues developed the theory of the demand primarily in the context of clinical psychological intervention aimed at individuals. In that context, the focus of interest is essentially on the subject's overall mode of relating to the world, thus on the semiotic level of highest abstraction and generalization that underlies that mode: affective symbolization (see, for example, Cordella et al., 2022) – affective self-other schemas, in the terminology of GTPI.

As mentioned previously, however, the demand that substantiates the client's request can also be represented on levels of lower abstraction. In what follows, we propose a map of the demand at the level of domain beliefs (see Chapter 3). We believe it is useful to do so because the map of the demand on this level of lower abstraction facilitates an understanding of the role that the demand and its analysis play in interventions at levels other than individual.

From the perspective we are adopting, the demand is a naïve theory substantiated by a network of beliefs that defines the order of things: the canon used to interpret events and nurture expectations about their evolution. More specifically, the network of beliefs that substantiates the demand underlying the client's request concerns:

- the explanation of the causes of the situation that is the subject of/motivates the request (hereafter: *problem conception*);
- the foreshadowing of the condition that the intervention is expected to achieve (hereafter: *goal conception*);
- the value that the goal has for the client (hereafter: *desirability conception*);
- the foreshadowing of what needs to happen for that condition to be accomplished (hereafter: *solution conception*);
- the expectation about what the professional is called upon to do to achieve what is desired (hereafter: *professional conception*);

- the idea about the level and form of involvement required of the client (hereafter: *client conception*);
- the idea about what kind of relationship and organizational agreements it makes sense to define and maintain with the professional (hereafter: *organization conception*).

Consider the following vignette. An executive of a small company that markets telephone products asks the psychologist for "a few hours of training" on effective communication to be supplied to its employees. The company – this is how the manager making the request justifies the request to the psychologist – has experienced a drop in productivity in recent months since the two top salespeople moved to another company. The manager would like the psychologist's training to provide employees with the communication tricks needed to be more convincing with potential buyers. The manager warns that the training will necessarily have to be held on a weekend, as it is not possible to suspend the company's activity during working hours. Table 5.1 summarizes the map of the demand underlying this request. In the right-hand column, we have included possible alternative beliefs, called out to highlight that the demand does not mirror a factual situation but one of the possible points of view from which the circumstances reported by the client may be interpreted. This means that the demand expresses the client's subjectivity (in this case, having the form of a specific organizational culture).

As can be seen, the reference of the demand largely overlaps the entire GTPI domain of interest – it represents its parallel at the level of the client's system of meaning. Just as the psychologist organizes her/his interpretation of the client's condition, the possible impact and desirability of her/his intervention, and the ways of regulating the relationship with the client, so does the client. What distinguishes the client's and the psychologist's systems of meaning is their different anchoring: the client's anchorage is common sense, mobilized through the language of desire; the psychologist anchors her/his system of meaning to scientific knowledge, characterized by the constraints that the language of theory and of method imposes on desire.

A final observation. The beliefs mapped previously are closely interconnected – for example, the client's idea about the resources (economic, organizational, symbolic) that it is canonical to invest in the intervention, as well as the expectation about the timeframe within which it is reasonable to expect results, depending on the conception of the problem, as well as on the conception of the goal and its desirability. As repeatedly pointed out, such beliefs are not autonomous "pieces" so much as elements of a single gestalt of abstract meaning – the conception of the problem, of the goal, of its desirability, and so on, are the projection on the plane closest to the experience of the client's view of the relationship with her/his world and the corresponding vision of how things work. This means that if, at the level of the discussion on which

TABLE 5.1 An example map of the demand

Belief	Content	Possible alternative content
Problem conception	Decline in productivity is due to sellers' inability to convince potential buyers	The drop in productivity reflects a change in the market of telephone products. The market decline reflects a latent conflict between the back office and sales personnel
Goal conception	Increased ability of salespeople to persuade customers	Development of a new market strategy and horizontal integration between business areas
Desirability conception	What is important is to make up for the drop in productivity	What is important is to use the critical event of productivity decline to understand how the environment with which the company interacts has evolved to design a development strategy that will remain sustainable over the medium term
Solution conception	Increasing the ability to convince potential customers depends on possessing communication tricks. To accomplish this, the solution is "a few hours" of training in effective communication	Increased sales ability depends on the ability to make sense of one's work and to understand and orient to the customer's point of view
Professional conception	The psychologist uses communication tricks to convince salespeople to motivate them and, at the same time, teach them so that they, in turn, convince their potential buyers	The psychologist supports the analysis of the impact of changes in the environment on the company and how the company can equip itself to deal with them
Client conception	Training should be carried out at a separate and additional time from organizational life. Training is about salespeople; it does not involve the rest of the company.	The psychologist's intervention is strategic, and therefore, it has to involve the organizational system as a whole
Organization conception	The relationship the client has with the psychologist serves to negotiate the operational details of the requested intervention. The manager does not expect to interact with the psychologist on the question underlying the request, as the latter is assumed to be self-evident	The relationship with the psychologist also involves the possibility of reasoning about the ideas the client has about the problems to be addressed and their solutions

our map is placed, such beliefs are treated as separate and interacting elements, this happens not because we recognize autonomy to such elements but because language imposes a limit on the possibility of accounting for the holistic organization of the system of meaning, forcing us to represent the latter through the approximation offered by the format of the description by interacting elements.

3 The governance of the client's request

The discussion proposed in the first section of this chapter should have highlighted how the psychological intervention (as well as any other type of professional intervention) can take different attitudes towards the client's request. More particularly, from the discussion previously, it follows that the psychologist's attitude can lie on a continuum, having at one end the view of the client's request as *given* and, at the other, the view of it as *to develop*.

We have seen that the interventions lying on the first side of the continuum are those that pursue goals and enact actions remaining within the constraints set by the client's demand. For example, consider a psychologist to whom the judge entrusts expert advice aimed at estimating the psychological damage suffered by a victim. In this case, the request defines the perimeter within which the psychologist's intervention is expected to move. Similarly, a psychologist in charge of a market research survey may deem it appropriate to produce her/his advice within the request that triggered its action. Interventions on the other side of the continuum, on the other hand, move in ways and purposes that are not immediately compatible with the canons of the request. Therefore, they need the request to be developed in order to make it compatible with the professional action. For instance, consider the case recalled in the previous chapter concerning the school principal's request that the psychologist meet students who had been exposed to their classmate's death as a result of an accident that occurred during normal school activities. In that situation, the psychologist hypothesized that in order to provide a useful response to the principal's request, it was more appropriate to have a meeting with teachers rather than with students. The agreement reached with the school principal on this mode of action is an example of the development of the request, consisting of a shift from the client's initial request.

It should be clear that the two ends of the continuum are ideal-typical abstractions. No intervention can operate by assuming the request as fully given. Similarly, all forms of meaning development are based on a shared premise of meaning between the practitioner and client system (see Chapter 4); consequently, the development of the request is always part of and sustained by a component of the demand that is taken for granted, as such operating as the basic premise of sense grounding the client-psychologist relationship.

The developmental space of the request

The development of the request can be exerted at different levels, which can be modeled in terms of two parameters.

The first parameter concerns the level of the demand where its change is pursued. We return here to the three levels on which we have articulated the vectors of intervention: empowerment, dialecticization, and deconstruction of meaning (see Chapter 4). Moving from the first to the third level, the governance of the request takes on a broader scope. An example of development of the request carried out at the level of empowerment is that provided by the psychologist, who specifies to the client the technical reasons why a particular sample design is necessary for the commissioned market survey. In doing so, the psychologist promotes a change in the request – the client accepts the technical specification and is willing to support the investment resulting from it. Returning to the case we referred to previously, the acquiescence gained by the school manager about the proposal to meet with teachers rather than students is an example of development of the request realized on the level of dialecticization, because it involves a change in the manager's implicit theory of the strategy to be adopted. An example of commissioning governance effected by the level of the deconstruction of meaning is reported by Carli and Paniccia (1999). A large company commissioned an advisory group to draft a program of personnel selection aimed at hiring motivated, reliable people willing to identify with the company. What the company expected was to find people with personality traits – motivation, availability, flexibility – such that they would be resources for the organization. The advisors engaged with the client in a detailed process of analysis and deconstruction of the demand grounding the request. One of the beliefs substantiating that demand that it was possible to deconstruct was the idea that human resource qualities reflect characteristics that are inherent to the individual rather than expressive of the way personnel and organizations interact with each other. This deconstruction enabled great growth in the client's investment in the intervention, which led the advisory group to serve for several years as global consultants supporting the company's human resource development policies.

The second parameter concerns the component of the intervention involved in the development of the request. More particularly, we propose distinguishing three components: *process, function*, and *use. Process* refers to the organization of the intervention (see Chapter 4). The development of the request related to the process concerns the agreement with the client on aspects that qualify the operation that the psychologist puts in place – for example, the agreement on a work program, parties involved, resources invested, timing, etc. This level of governance of the client's request is essential; in many cases, it is the first necessary step, both to create the conditions for the intervention and as the preliminary stage for further developments of the request. On this point, let us return to the case of the school principal who asked the psychologist to meet with students, to whom the psychologist counter-proposed meeting with teachers. In this case, the development of the request is about the process. At the same time, however, this development was the way to promote further development related to the *function*: to shift the goal pursued by the psychologist from fostering the students' elaboration of the traumatic experience to promoting the teachers' skills in addressing the critical situation. Thus, in the case of the function, the development of the request involves its objective – namely, the function of the psychologist and its intervention. Consider, for example, a patient who comes to the psychotherapist for a specific problem – a symptom – and, in the course of the clinical work, expands the meaning of the treatment so that they come to see the psychotherapy as the way to improve their overall ability to make sense of their life. By *use*, the third component, we mean the process through which the client generates utility from the output of the intervention (see Section 6). In this case, what the development of the request aims for is the client's ability to valorize what the intervention is able to produce. Let us return to the case reported by Carli and Paniccia (1999), mentioned previously. The big company's request developed on the level of process – for example, advisors and the client agreed on a work program of considerably greater magnitude than initially envisioned by the request – as well as on that of the function – the client agreed with the psychologists as to the utility of redefining the function of personnel selection as aimed at innovating the corporate organizational culture, rather than identifying people with desirable personality traits. However, the peculiar aspect of the development of the request, in this case, was on the level of the use – the company invested a significant amount of resources (organizational, symbolic, economic) to promote and manage the inner organizational environment in order to optimize the innovative impact on the new human resources in accordance with the criteria agreed with the advisors. For example, the company undertook to analyze the contexts of the location of the new personnel, train mentors to whom to entrust the newly hired in the insertion phase, offer supervision services to support this function, and monitor and verify the insertion phase. As a result of the development of the client's request, which occurred on the level of use, the intervention changed its face radically – from an action of personnel selection to that of an intervention of global organizational development.

The combination of the two parameters presented in the previous section allows us to trace what we call the *space of development of the request* (Figure 5.1). The two dimensions of the space are not independent. As the examples proposed in the previous section should have made clear, it is legitimate to assume that the more the development of the request is pursued in strategic terms (i.e., from bottom to top along the vertical axis of Figure 5.1), the more interventions aimed at promoting far-reaching

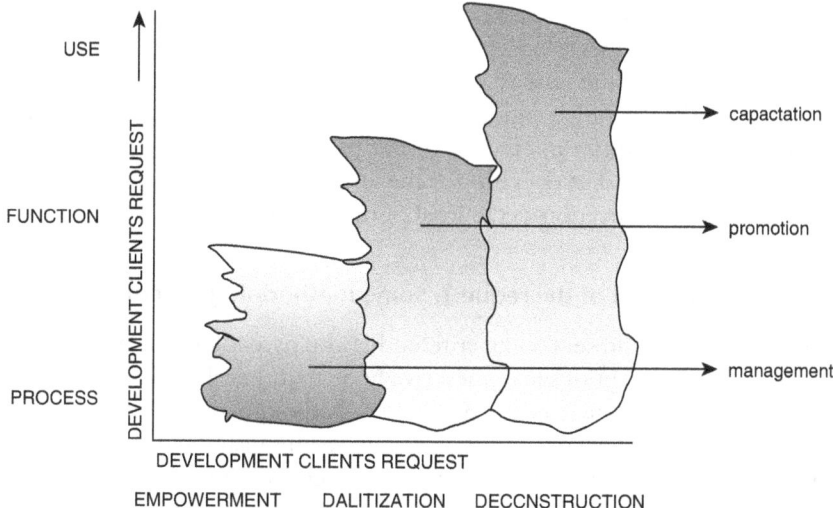

FIGURE 5.1   The development space of the client's request

changes in meaning (from left to right along the horizontal axis of the figure) are needed.

Because of this, we have identified three levels of development of the request (darker parts of the figure). The first level – *management* – is about the maintenance of the client's request or its modulation. It mainly concerns the process. Vectors of empowerment (Chapter 4) find their utility at this level mainly. The second level – *promotion* – has as its center of gravity the function of the psychologist, the revision and/or expansion of the intervention's expected output. To this end, vectors of empowerment need to be supplemented with operations covered by the vectors of dialecticization, aimed at changing the beliefs on which the client's idea about the solution to be pursued is based and, thus, the function that the consultant should fulfill in that perspective. The third level is that of *capacitation*. As the example taken up by Carli and Paniccia showed, in this case, what changes is not so much what is expected of the consultant but the client's competence, her/his ability to valorize the impact of the output; consequently, what changes is the very meaning of the intervention, as a result of the deconstruction of the client's demand (in the example: from personnel selection to promotion of organizational development).

A final note. As Figure 5.1 highlights, the three levels now outlined – management, promotion, and capacitation – are nested within each other. This means that the level of higher momentum can be interpreted as an evolution of the level of lower momentum. On the methodological level, this implies a circularity in the governance of the client's request: on the one hand, the development of the request tends to move from less to more complex levels – with the former used as preparatory to the latter; on the other hand, the development of the request at the level of function and use results in an evolution of the operative conditions of intervention. For example, a dialecticization of the request in relation to the process may be the premise for a subsequent development operating at the level of function, which in turn may produce further innovation at the level of management.

4 The development of the request. Some methodological criteria

In this section, we present some criteria that the psychologist can use to promote the development of the request (we hope that the labels we have enjoyed giving the criteria will help in that sense). Although these criteria are also designed to convey a change in meaning, we distinguish them from the intervention vectors presented in the previous chapter. This is for two reasons: first, while the vectors are functions that we have described in terms of the function they pursue, the criteria for the development of the request presented in what follows consist of logical rules and operational modes that organize the use of the vectors in the context of the governance of the request; second, unlike the vectors, which can be used in both the operational and organizational components of the intervention, the criteria are specifically focused on the latter, and in particular on the context of elaboration of the client's request.

The client system

With the (partial) exception of interventions that target individuals, the psychologist's professional action involves the involvement of a plurality of actors. In what follows, we will use the term *client system* (or, more briefly, client) to refer to the entire network of actors involved in the intervention. Within the client system, it is appropriate to distinguish different subsystems of actors (which can be either individuals or groups associated with organizational functions), each corresponding to a functional position within the intervention organization: *contractors, recipients, beneficiaries, third parties,* and *stakeholders*.

- contractors are the actors who exercise decisional power over the intervention, its activation, as well as the forms of its regulation and conclusion;
- recipients are the subjects to whom the psychologist's action is directed and in relation to whom the immediate result of the intervention is determined;
- beneficiaries are the subjects to whom the impact that the intervention is intended to generate is aimed. In other words, regardless of their direct participation in the intervention, they determine its value, that is, the translation of its immediate result into a form of utility (see Section 6);

- third parties are the actors who, regardless of their being part of the recipients or beneficiaries, play a role in the organizational process that conveys and regulates professional actions;
- stakeholders are additional actors in the intermediate space between the client system and its environment. They deserve to be considered part of the intervention's client system because the impact it generates is a source of utility for them. In other words, the impact of the intervention impacts their field of action and interest.

To clarify the typology proposed, let us refer to the two interventions we mentioned previously. The school principal and the top managers of the human resources area are the contractors; teachers met by the psychologist and the personnel who underwent the selection are the recipients; students and the company's business areas of placement of the hired personnel are beneficiaries; the school support staff who kept open the school office to enable the psychologist to meet teachers and the staff of the large company involved in the administrative management of the intervention are examples of third parties; and finally, families of the students and clients of the large company are examples of stakeholders.

The wide-angle rule

The map of the client system enables us to highlight two relevant points concerning the development of the request. First, actors of the client system may locate themselves in more than one of the positions of the typology proposed at the same time. In addition, this geography of locations may change over time, also as a result of the intervention. For example, in the intervention with the big company, the business areas of placement of the hired personnel began the intervention as beneficiaries and turned into recipients, too. Second, the request does not coincide with the action of the contractor; indeed, as intended here (see Section 2.1), each actor involved in the intervention, by reason of the position assumed in it and its own project, enacts a form of engagement with the psychologist's action (e.g., from full cooperation to rejection), and in doing so partakes in the dynamic construction and implementation of the request. Accordingly, the request must be conceived as a field of forces – henceforth: the *request field*. This gives rise to the utility of mapping the whole network of commitments in its varying intensity and direction, both among the different actors involved in the intervention and over time. The wide-angle lens rule lies in this – it is appropriate that the dynamic representation of the investment can be accomplished in a manner similar to how a photographer uses such a lens to encompass the entire field of vision in a single glance.

The judoka rule

The request field is not homogeneous. Each subject participates in the intervention with its own project, reflecting the part of the contextual system meaning in which it is embedded. The more complex the client system, the more heterogeneous is the request field. A client system composed of a parent and an adolescent designated as a patient describes an already sufficiently complex field where the two requests cannot be taken for granted as aligned. One can, therefore, imagine how differentiated the request field of a large company, a public administration, or a school may be. Such fields reproduce within the intervention strategies, interests, conflicts, networks of power, and communication – in short, local cultures – that animate the life of the client system. Request fields like that must be mapped so that they can be taken appropriately into account in the design and governance of the intervention. The criterion at stake is that the intervention must provide a representation within itself (usually in organizational terms, namely at the level of objectives, roles, and devices deployed) to the relevant actors and requests that are active within the request field. The ostrich policy is thus a loser – leaving the conflicting power groups of the client system out of the intervention does not free it from them. On the contrary, the only way to be able to govern them so as to limit their centrifugal impact is to allow them a voice within the intervention. Imagine, for example, that the relationship between the top management of the human resources development division on which the personnel selection policy depends and a business area where some of the selected resources are expected to be placed is marked by a deep conflict rooted in the different view of the area's functions. Representing this conflict within the intervention is achieved by arranging devices that enable the intervention to treat it as a source of knowledge and regulation of action-for example, by setting the analysis of the processes of the placement of the resource in the business areas as one of the relevant issues subject to joint monitoring by the advisor and the top management. By doing so, the consultant can try to govern the critical fallout that conflict might produce on the intervention. The alternative – keeping the conflict outside the boundaries of the intervention – would not prevent its effects from occurring while limiting the possibilities of managing them. In this respect, the psychologist operates like the judoka, who – rather than trying to resist the opponent's movement – uses their own body as a lever in order to exploit the opponent's movement to their advantage. Similarly, the psychologist arranges devices – levers that do not serve to protect the intervention from conflict but allow it to be represented within the intervention and, thanks to that, within the limits of what is possible and necessary to elaborate/channel it with towards the purposes of the professional action.

The bus rule

This criterion is a corollary of the previous one. As already noted, the request field is not homogeneous. Organizational theory has pointed out that socio-technical structures are inherently plural (Bonazzi, 1989). Differently from the functionalist paradigm, social action is not achieved through the sharing of goals and interests; rather, it is produced *in spite of* the inherent conflict between actors (Crozier & Friedberg, 1977), thanks to superordinate systems that nonetheless make some degree of cooperation preferable. From this perspective, the intervention does not assume that the actors involved pursue the same goals. On the contrary, it assumes that each subject pursues its own project and expresses its own agenda of interests and priorities. This means that cooperation within the inherently plural request field is not to be sought on the level of identifying common elements – namely, in terms of sharing. Rather, it is to be pursued in terms of *compatibility*, that is to say, in terms of defining sufficiently abstract perspectives of purpose such that they are representable by the different actors as compatible, and thus functional, to their project. Elsewhere, one of us has called this form of cooperation *reciprocity* (Cremaschi et al., 2021). In the reciprocity model, actors do not share the same goal; each pursues their own idiosyncratic interest; at the same time, action is organized in such a way that each actor pursues their own interest through processes whose realization requires other actors to pursue their own goals. Thus, cooperation in the form of reciprocity is systemic in nature: it does not depend on the exchange that takes place exclusively at the level between actors, i.e., on what they identify as a common element; rather, it is a superordinate framework that establishes cooperation as a functional mode that each actor adopts to pursue its own project. To conceive of intervention in terms of reciprocity is to assume that the psychologist does not seek organic convergence within and with the request field. Rather, he operates like the driver of a regular bus, picking up passengers who have idiosyncratic purposes, which the bus route includes within a framework of compatibility. One way to operate in this direction is to define superordinate criteria that can be used by different actors to define consensuality scenarios. Such criteria do not define a commonality of purpose or action among actors but participation in a common cognitive and/or decision-making procedure. Consensus is thus about the process rather than the output. For example, the psychologist discusses with the recipients a package of proposals previously negotiated with the contractor from which to identify the working solution that, from their perspective, is most useful and consistent with their views and goals.

The rule of decomposition

This criterion aims to illustrate a way to engage with the request in terms of compatibility. As we have noted previously (Chapters 2 and 3), the premise of sense that grounds the request (i.e., the demand) can be broken down into components, similar to what happens with a molecule that can be decomposed in its atomic components. On this basis, the psychologist can focus the conflict on one of the components and use the others instead to substantiate the compatibility framework with the client system. Let us return to the conversation that took place between the psychologist and the school principal who requested an intervention in the students' class. The psychologist made a breakdown of the premise of sense underlying such a request, identifying the following dimensions as relevant: a) a fatal incident that occurred during school time has a catastrophic traumatic impact on the school, b) students are the first and most affected by such an impact, c) it is the school's job to help students, and d) helping students requires an outside professional to enter directly into a relationship with them. The psychologist welcomes the first three components and on the basis of the consensus thus defined, proposed a dialecticization of the fourth component, stating that to help students does not necessarily mean one needs to relate to them directly.

The Chinese rule

Confucius is credited with the proverb, "Sit by the riverbank and wait; sooner or later you will see the corpse of your enemy pass by." Now, the request is not the enemy, but the other position of the client system in the dialectic with which the space of intervention is construed. The development of the request is, therefore, both a cooperative and a conflictual relationship: the client brings otherness, and the intervention is ultimately the process of conflictual cooperation with this alterity. What the proverb highlights is that this process must be thought of in terms of temporality – as an evolution that proceeds in steps, usually in incremental terms, sometimes in leaps. Conceiving the development of the request in terms of temporality has several implications beyond the obvious one of having the patience to wait for the maturation times that characterize any process. It means thinking of it as a resource that is never acquired but that has to be constantly monitored, consolidated, and built upon in the course of the intervention. It means, moreover, representing the organizational component of the intervention as operating systematically, intertwined with the operational component; in other words, not only thinking of the development of the request as a preliminary and propaedeutic stage of the intervention but also, conversely, considering the intervention as a way for the further development of the request. A final implication: thinking of the request in temporal terms leads to organizing what is done at a given moment in the intervention by taking into account not only its current meaning within the request field but also how it may be reinterpreted at a later time because of the further developed of the request. For example, consider the psychologist who, in the initiation phase of the interventions, proposes to the client to schedule a follow-up meeting to be held at the conclusion. The psychologist is aware that at the time he puts forward the proposal, it may be considered marginal by the client; however, he makes the assumption that when the follow-up meeting takes place, the level of investment achieved by the client will allow for full exploitation of this device.

Murphy's rule

This criterion is a corollary of the previous one. As just noted, the request field tends to decay in the sense that if left to itself, it tends to be assimilated and, therefore, reshaped by the culture of the client system. It is, therefore, useful to provide, as with automobiles, a program of periodic revision of the request field, along with constant monitoring of possible weak signals of its decay over the course of the intervention. From a complementary point of view, it is good for the psychologist to assume, like Murphy, that if things can go wrong, they will. This, of course, is not to wallow in pessimism but, on the contrary, to plan ex-ante for the devices and procedures useful for managing critical issues that may emerge in the request field. Governing the crisis requires resources that, by definition, are not available at the time of the crisis and, therefore, must be identified when the conditions for doing so are available. An example of such a device is when the psychotherapist, at the time of the initial definition of the contract, agrees with the patient that, should the patient wish to quit the work in progress, this will be discussed beforehand in the session. Another example related to larger-scale interventions is the establishment of a steering committee to which to entrust, among other functions, the addressing of critical issues that may arise in the unfolding of the intervention.

The rubber band rule

As repeatedly noted, the relationship between psychologist and client is inherently conflictual in that consultant and client systems carry necessarily different views and interests. On the other hand, conflict is not synonymous with competition – intervention is not a zero-sum game where the victory of one means the defeat of the other. The conflict comprising intervention is the condition and form of carrying it out. However, to be productive, the conflict must be kept within appropriate levels. These levels cannot be defined once and for all and in absolute terms: they depend on the stability of the working alliance between the psychologist and client system. Therein lies the rule of the rubber band: the psychologist imprints on their action the maximum degree of otherness that the relationship with the client can tolerate – they will stretch the rubber band as far as possible, but without taking it beyond the breaking point. In the clinical field, the rubber band rule is implicit in the emphasis placed on the therapeutic alliance (e.g., Lingiardi, 2002) – the firmer the alliance, the more the therapist can move the focus of their own interventions from the peripheral to the nuclear areas of the patient's self-system. From a different point of view, the rubber band rule harks back to the Vygotskyian concept of the zone of proximal development: the interaction between the client's and the psychologist's systems of meaning allows for development to the extent that the latter is both sufficiently innovative and sufficiently proximal to the client's system of meaning.

The car battery rule

This criterion is complementary to the previous one. The operational component of the intervention increases the conflict between psychologist and client, as it exposes the latter to the otherness that professional action brings with it. As widely recognized by clinicians and researchers concerned with the psychotherapeutic process, the relationship between professional and client proceeds as a continuous alternation of moments of rupture and reparation of the working alliance (Safran & Muran, 2000). On the one hand, as seen (rubber band rule), this implies keeping the conflict within the margins of compatibility of the relationship with the client system; on the other hand, it requires taking into account that professional action needs to be constantly nurtured by the working alliance, i.e., by the client's commitment to it. Therein lies the analogy with the car battery: the intervention, just because it is conducted, keeps the battery-working alliance that serves to power the whole apparatus charged. Several operations are available in the clinical literature that respond to the purpose of strengthening the working alliance – e.g., empathic mirroring, encouragement, and the assumption of a nonjudgmental listening attitude. Some of these operations can also be used on larger-scale interventions. On the other hand, it is difficult to think that one can promote a working alliance with a public administrator or top manager by relying exclusively or even primarily on empathic mirroring and encouragement. At the levels of intervention on which the request field has collective actors as protagonists, the client system investment in intervention requires drivers of institutional and strategic nature, that is, modalities that operate at the level of the power and interest relations of the actors of the field. Two of the principles proposed by Jason (2013), already referred to in Chapter 3, are examples of these kinds of drivers: identifying who has the power to influence the processes related to the problem being addressed by the intervention and creating coalitions with community actors who share what the intervener aims for. As can be seen, these two criteria highlight the role that stakeholders can play in developing the request field.

Fabrizio's rule

This criterion is a generalization of the previous one. In one of his most beautiful songs, "Tito's last Will," the Italian songwriter Fabrizio De André rereads the Ten Commandments from the point of view of Titus, the thief crucified beside Jesus[1]. The psychologist should operate similarly to the songwriter – to move according to their own criteria, based on the knowledge provided by scientific psychology but at the same time have systematic awareness of the fact that the client, like Titus, enters a relationship with the intervention in the terms and by reason of his own standpoint of subjectivity (beliefs, interests, projects). And if such a standpoint is capable of rewriting the ten commandments, we can imagine what overturning the criteria proposed by the psychologist is capable of. Making the clients' point of view compatible requires, first of all, recognizing its autonomy, in the fact that it cannot be reduced to and disciplined by the scientific evidence. More generally, as noted about the judoka rule, to act as if the client's point of view were not active – or at any rate was neutralizable on the basis of the normativity of the scientific knowledge underlying the intervention – has the sole effect of turning it into a kind of loose cannon, an uncontrolled source of destabilization of the intervention.

The rule of the sculptor

The development of the client's request can be thought of as a dynamic of progressive focalization: a process of recursive accumulation of constraints that increasingly increases the area of compatibility between psychologist and client system. It is in this sense that the psychologist proceeds like the sculptor – working to reduce the variability of the relationship with the client, as does the sculptor who subtracts, progressively and recursively, parts from the block of matter so that a form emerges from it. The validity of this mode goes beyond the psychological intervention. In what has become a classic of that field of study, a political scientist (Lindblom, 1959) theorized something similar to the sculptor's rule as a general principle of policy-making – to proceed by subsequent approximations (*muddling through*). According to the author, public policies are not realized as the execution of a plan exhaustively defined upstream of the intervention. On the contrary, policies proceed incrementally, step by step, contingently established, and based on existing constraints. In other words, policy-making continuously adapts the formal plan to circumstances and moves by successive approximations aimed at improving what has been done previously, which in turn is open to subsequent adjustment. We return in this regard to the development of the client's request reported by Carli and Paniccia (1999). We have summarized its initial and final points. The process actually lasted several years (the Chinese rule) and proceeded as the recursive introduction of successive constraints in the relationship with the client – for example, it was initially agreed that personnel selection criteria should be anchored in the company's lines of development. Later, the constraint was introduced to interpret this development in terms of changing organizational culture. This created the conditions for introducing as a further constraint the unsuitability of conceiving the hired resources in a *vacuum* and the consequent need to govern the process of insertion in the corporate location, and so on, until the stabilization of the meaning of the intervention as a global strategic advisor in support of the company's development.

The Manzonian shouting rule

Besides being useless, it is counterproductive to solicit the client to take responsibility for an impossible task. Intervention must avoid following the example of the Spanish ruler of Milan described in Manzoni's *The Betrothed*, who issued edicts that the harsher and more restrictive they were, the less they were respectable and respected. It is not enough for actors involved in the intervention to express their consent about the manner, timing, and content of their participation in the intervention. It is also necessary that what is agreed upon could be realistically actionable and that any disregard of agreements could be manageable – that is, it could leave a trace in the organization of the intervention and can thus be elaborated. Otherwise, the normative structure of the intervention takes on an aura of falsity – what has been established is not only incapable of regulating the relationship between psychologist and client system but ends up being emptied of functional meaning and acquiring a merely ritualistic value. For example, in the context of a research/intervention entrusted to the psychologist by a community health service, the participation of a group of junior researchers (third parties) had been planned, with the role of conducting interviews with a large sample of the local population. The contract with these resources included detailed standards and technical specifications of the assignment given to them. After an initial moment of enthusiastic adherence to the work plan put forward by the psychologist, the first signs of the weakening of the junior researchers' commitment began to emerge: a weakening that ran through the group as a whole, interpretable, among other things, as a reaction of conflict with the community service. Faced with this dynamic, the psychologist considered it counterproductive to invoke the normative datum of the contract. Doing so would have activated a device in that context of limited regulatory capacity, further emptying it of functionality; at the same time, it would have prevented the identification of more effective forms of regulation of the area of the request field associated with this client subsystem. The psychologist, therefore, decided to discuss with the junior researchers a redefinition of their tasks, compatible with the requirements of the intervention and, at the same time, consistent with their desire to see the reasons for their conflict with the community service recognized (see the bus rule).

The cat rule (not to tell)

This criterion is related to the previous one. One risk any intervention runs is to confuse the objective pursued with the ways to accomplish it. In many circumstances, the line between these two aspects is blurred, and in any case is always to be defined contingently by reason of circumstances. Consider a situation of conflict among actors: is the proposal of having the actors involved in the conflict to meet and negotiate a means or the result to be pursued? If there are conditions for this to happen profitably, then it is a means, but if those conditions are not there, then it is a goal. A famous Italian soccer coach – Giovanni Trapattoni – used to repeat a phrase that has become a cult favorite – "Don't say cat if you don't have it in the sack." This is what we suggest that the psychologist also has to do: do not assume as established the compatibility of the request field just on the basis of the formal agreement expressed by the actors involved. Such compatibility has to be monitored and construed, not just assumed or required of the client system.

5 The analysis of the demand

Although some of the criteria of development of the client's request outlined in the previous section (e.g., system-client, Chinese rule) have cross-cutting validity, overall, they focus on the levels of development that we have previously defined as *management* and *promotion*. Indeed, as we have observed, the capacitation level involves a change of broader scope: the increase of the competence of the client to use the output of the intervention. The change of meaning in the case in question takes on a reflexive valence – to change is not so much just a belief related to the object but the client's project of using the results of the intervention. In the previous chapter (Chapter 4), we connected this type of change to the deconstructive type vectors (performative interpretation and structuring). We consider the *analysis of demand* (Carli, 1987a, 1987b, 1993; Carli & Paniccia, 2003) the function of the intervention that deploys these deconstructive vectors in the context and for the purpose of developing the client's request at the level of use.

The structural incompetence of the client

In order to understand the role that the analysis of the demand plays within the development of the client's request, it is appropriate to consider an element that is peculiar to the request for psychological intervention. Indeed, in the case of psychological intervention, *the client's premise of sense comprising the demand tends to overlap with the premise of sense that feeds the criticality the client copes with.*

A point already discussed crops up again here (see Chapter 2). According to the psycho-semiotic perspective we are using, psychological intervention fulfills the function of promoting the client's ability to produce interpretations appropriate to their project. This means that the client who turns to the psychologist, by definition, has a system of meaning that demands being developed.

However, the client possesses only one system of meaning; consequently, the request cannot but be based on the same system of meaning that underlies the criticality with which the client intends to cope. Ultimately, in the case of psychology, *a linkage can be established between the criticality of the interpretation and the interpretation of the criticality.* Consider the following examples. Take a man immersed in a persecutory and malignant view of the world, which nurtures a suspicious, aggressive, and recriminatory attitude running through his close relations as well as his social and professional engagements. Such a stance has compromised the man's quality of life, his ability to establish stable and rewarding interpersonal relationships, and his ability to achieve meaningful results at work. Following yet another failure, the person decides to consult a psychologist. His approach to the professional does not deviate from the script. Convinced that the psychologist's only motivation for meeting him is to use him for his own interests, he spends the first few encounters seeking confirmation of his expectation that he is confronted with yet another specimen of the malignity of the world he constantly experiences. Another example. The teachers of a classroom regard the school's reputation as a core value and believe that it depends primarily on good relations with students' families. On that basis, they have developed an increasingly submissive attitude over the years, aimed at pandering to parents' expectations and requests. This has resulted in a progressive renunciation of exercising those components of the teaching activity that are potentially in conflict with family expectations and requests addressed to the school – year after year, workloads for students have been reduced, evaluation criteria relaxed, disciplinary measures ritualized, etc. All this has generated in the faculty a widespread feeling of ineffectiveness, disaffection, and loss of meaning, symptomatically expressed by the numerous transfer requests and outbreaks of conflict among colleagues. Teachers turn to the psychologist – the concern motivating them is that problems they are experiencing within their group may jeopardize the school's reputation. They expect the psychologist to focus on the vicissitudes of their group, as this is what they consider critical. They react with veiled disappointment to the psychologist's proposal to explore what is happening in the relationship with students and families. A last example. A public administrator, as part of his duties, is called upon to promote the social use of some land assets confiscated from organized crime. His idea is that the valorization of these assets is a matter to be managed in economic-managerial terms through the promotion of a youth managerial lever that, with the appropriate financial support, includes the territorial assets in circuits of production and services that are sustainable in the long run. On that basis, he asks the psychologist to conduct a series of training courses to promote entrepreneurial and managerial skills for those who have to manage the assets. The administrator envisions the courses as aimed at providing participants with leadership and team management skills.

Let us see what these three examples have in common. In all three cases, the actor conveying the request – the contractor – is in a relationship with reality through and in terms of the mediation of a project. In the first example, the project is global and concerns the whole existential domain of the patient – experiencing stable and rewarding relationships within which to achieve meaningful social and professional results; in the second and third cases, the project concerns a specific domain related to the function that the contractors exercise – the improvement of the school activity, the valorization of confiscated assets, respectively. In all three cases, the project is based on – and at the same time finds its constraint in – an interpretation of the situation the contractor has to cope with: the persecutory and malignant view of the world, the good reputation of the school among families as a core value, the economic nature of the problems related to the social valorization of the assets confiscated from organized crime. The project is thus pursued on this interpretive basis: in terms of a generalized recriminatory and aggressive attitude in the first case, of the adoption of a compliant and ritualized mode of relating to families in the second case, and in the choice of using youth entrepreneurship as a decisive lever in the third case. The three examples imply that such ways of pursuing projects are problematic, and thus, the interpretation that underlies them should be understood as a constraint on the subjects' possibilities of entering fruitful relationships with the world. In this lies the *criticality of interpretation.* This is clearly evident in the case of the man animated by a persecutory view of reality; however, it can also be grasped in the other two cases. The passive pandering of the families' expectations results in an emptying of the teachers' function; above all, the interpretation that underlies it leaves no room for the possibility of exploring further models of relationship with families, capable of basing cooperation on the valorization of the intrinsic dialectic that exists between the institutional mission of the school and the educational demand of lifeworlds (Salvatore & Scotto di Carlo, 2005). Similarly, the economic/managerial interpretation of the valorization of the confiscated goods backgrounds the cultural context that mediates the relationship between the community and these goods – it treats goods in an instrumental key, as if they were mere material objects, without considering their symbolic value – the fact that they are *goods confiscated from organized crime* and as such involve the local population. Ultimately, to paraphrase Freud, the three client systems *suffer from solutions.* The request they propose to the psychologist reflects this criticality; in all three cases, the interpretation that fuels the criticality also grounds the request and, therefore, makes it critical as well. The man enters a relationship with the psychologist as if the latter were yet another manifestation of the persecutory and malignant world; the teachers expect the psychologist to relate to them according to the same principle of compliance that they adopt as the canon of their own actions; the public administrator prefigures the psychologist's contribution because of an instrumental conception of managerial and entre-preneurial skills and their promotion not unlike that which organizes the pro-ject of valorization of confiscated property. In all three cases, the *interpretation of the criticality* – the demand – that grounds and configures the commission reflects/reproduces the criticality of the interpretation.

Ultimately, the client of the psychological intervention can be recognized as *structurally incompetent* (Salvatore, 2016a) in the sense that the client reproduces in the request addressed to the psychologist the system of meaning – and the premise of sense at its core – that fuels the criticality that the relation-ship itself is called upon to address (Figure 5.2).

The structural incompetence of the psychologist's client is a peculiarity of the psychological intervention. Obviously, whatever profession is involved, the request is incompetent by definition. As noted previously, if the patient who turns to the practitioner were able to diagnose the condition from which they are suffering and identify the appropriate treatment, they would not need the practitioner. We turn to the professional because we are incompetent as to the state of affairs we entrust to the professional. Inevitably, the charge that clients direct to the professional is affected by the incompetence with which they interpret the condition that motivates it. The authors of this book know a practitioner that, some time ago, saved himself from a serious cardiac crisis because his knowledge in the field enabled him to recognize the warning signs of the event, enabling him to arrive at the emergency room in time. Such a level of expertise in the request can only be achieved if one has sufficient medi-cal knowledge. If our friend had been a talented expert in botany, we would probably have one less friend today. In general, in the case of the other pro-fessions, the incompetence of the client's request concerns the interpretation of the problem and/or the contribution of the expert, and it may affect the

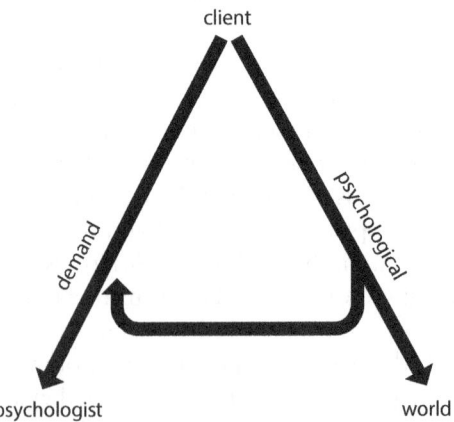

FIGURE 5.2 Relationship between customer meaning system and demand

relationship with the professional. The issues of adherence to medical care are a paradigmatic example of the client's incompetence. One of us realized how much expertise, commitment, and technical resources it requires to design and implement sound only when he got to enter such a world through his own son's work. Until then, if he had ever commissioned sound for some event, he would have considered costs and production time roughly equivalent to those required to get a coffee at the bar. In the case of the other professions, however, *the incompetence of the client is not associated with/empowered by the criticality that motivates it.* In fact, the criticality that motivates the request in the case of other professions is configured as relating to factors other than the dynamic of sensemaking; consequently, the system of meaning that substantiates the request is not related to criticality. The buyer of a property may be convinced that notaries are of no use (incompetent request); however, this belief in no way relates to the fact that the notarial deed is the form necessary to give legal value to the transfer of ownership of the property (the problem/purpose that motivates the request). Similarly, the naïve belief that the client possesses about the static problem plaguing their apartment may influence the relationship with the engineer – for example, the more serious the problem is deemed to be, the greater the willingness to invest in consulting – but it certainly has no relation to the static of the building.

We thus arrive at a conclusion. In the case of psychology, the request exhibits a fractal form: it reproduces in itself the client's system of meaning and, thus, its critical valence, the one on which the intervention is called to operate. This means that the client of the intervention lends itself to be conceptualized as structurally incompetent – that is to say, incompetent not because this or that client may interpret the problem inappropriately; but insofar as there is an intrinsic commensality between the meaning that generates the problem and the meaning that organizes the request that the client addresses to the psychologist. Because of this, psychological intervention has an interest in not taking the client's request for granted and in valorizing its difference from the scientific knowledge foundational to the psychologist's action. We do not propose such valorization as an absolute necessity of the intervention; rather, we see it as an opportunity: a methodological function of the psychological intervention that enhances the psychologist's ability to access the client's system of meaning, ultimately, her/his subjectivity-in-action.

Analysis of the demand and development of the client's request. Some examples

We devote this section to presenting a few examples chosen to cover a plurality of levels on which psychological intervention can act.

In the case of intervention on the individual, the analysis of demand overlaps substantially with the analysis of the transferential-countertransferential dynamic that configures the intersubjective field of the psychologist-client relationship. With reference to psychotherapy, Carli (1987b) considers the analysis of the demand to be a form of early analysis of the transference – *prototransfer analysis*, according to the terminology he used – which extends the analysis of the relationship between psychotherapist and patient to the affective interpretation that the latter constructs of psychotherapy and of the act of making it the object of the request. In other words, the analysis of the demand treats the relationship between psychologist and client not only in its interpersonal dimension but also in its socio-institutional component, i.e., the socio-cultural premise of sense that organizes the client's request of psychotherapy, even before the interpersonal exchange with the clinician that the psychotherapy mediates.

Let us return to the case presented in Chapter 3. Mr. D. approached the psychologist because of his feeling of being annihilated by his wife's emotional estrangement. In the first meetings, he spoke of his anguish over his wife's attitude toward him. He did not express to the psychologist an idea of how he thought the latter could help him: the meaning and targeting of his request seemed self-evident to him, coinciding with his state of suffering. The psychologist hypothesized that this attitude was the performative sign of an interpretation of psychotherapy as an ideal totalizing object, which, by receiving/containing the client, constituted the solution to everything. This hypothesis helped in understanding the content of the request – presenting Mr. D.'s pain to the psychotherapist was tantamount to communicating a desire for psychotherapy to take charge of him in its entirety, not unlike someone who goes to the emergency room complaining of chest pain and believing that this state of need is sufficient to mobilize the medical staff to take charge. The analysis of the demand thus enabled the psychologist to understand from the very first moments of the encounter with the patient the latter's propensity to consider himself the bearer of a self-representation as totally in need of the other, similar to a child who feels safe only in the arms of the parent. Understanding such a pattern of interpretation helped the psychologist to carry out three operations. First, formulate an initial hypothesis about the problems the patient was encountering in his relationship with the significant dimensions of his world, including his wife. More specifically, the hypothesis was that Mr. D. interpreted as radical criticality the circumstances in which, within significant relationships, his absolutized desire to be taken care of did not find satisfaction. This situation was evidently fostered as much by the rigidity of Mr. D.'s expectation as by the other's reaction to that expectation. Second, to develop Mr. D.'s request relative to a work plan centered on the vicissitudes of the marital relationship, but nonetheless expanded to include other life situations that exhibited the same issue, albeit with less significant impact. This development of the request (at the level of process and function) was accomplished essentially through a series of dialecticizations, carried out by the psychologist through the proposal, made as early as the first interview, to explore other areas of the patient's life in order to compare what was happening in them with what had been said about the relationship with his wife. Finally, the proposal of an explicit representation of Mr. D.'s demand to him – expressed with the metaphor of the other as a perfect mother to whom he could be totally entrusted – served as an anchor of the subsequent explorations that took place during the long psychotherapeutic journey that followed the first interviews reported here, and the outcomes of which were partly mentioned in Chapter 3 (for a discussion related to the link between analysis of the demand and early analysis of the transference-countertransference dynamic, see Salvatore et al., submitted).

Let us return to the case of the large company commissioning an intervention of personnel selection, described by Carli and Paniccia (1999), as an example of analysis of the demand exercised in the relationship with a client expressed by an organizational system. As mentioned previously, the requester (the head of the personnel area of the company) had asked the advisory group of psychologists to select individuals with a personality profile deemed desirable. The advisors took up this request by involving the client in a complex process of understanding and elaboration of the premises grounding the request. This process took place partly prior to the intervention in ad hoc seminars addressed to management and partly during the course of the intervention with periodic meetings with key actors of the client system. In the context of this process, it was possible for psychologists and client to agree that the initial request was based on the assumption – i.e., the demand – that personnel selection serves to identify people with certain personality traits, valuable in their own right (people who are motivated, helpful, etc.). Thanks to these qualities, once they were placed in the workplace, the newly hired personnel would be able to identify themselves as resources for the company. The deconstruction of this premise enabled the elaboration of innovative meanings. We recall here, in particular, two of them: a) the idea that the organizational value of the personnel to be selected is not contained in the individual but depends on the interaction between the actors and the company's development goals and, therefore, on the related projects of valorization of human resources, and b) the idea that the ability of the new personnel to operate as a resource for the company depends significantly on how the company governs the relationship with them, with particular attention to the phase of initial inclusion. We suggest the development of these two meanings as an instance of change in meaning that is at the level we have called structural transformation (Chapter 3). These two meanings, in fact, qualify the client's premise of sense through three dimensions of meaning, which were not present in the initial form of the demand: 1) the dimension of the company's strategic investment in its future – it is this dimension of meaning that makes it thinkable that human resources are not chosen because of a given characteristic, but because of a strategic purpose; 2) the dimension of contextuality – because of which it became thinkable that the value of human resources is not an immanent characteristic of the person but of their relationship with the context; and 3) the dimension of the evolutive co-construction of value, which makes it possible to think that the value of the human resources depends on how the company governs the relationship between the organizational environment and personnel over time, starting from the first stage of inclusion. The emergence of these innovative meanings enabled a significant qualitative and quantitative development in the client, the contents of which we have previously highlighted (see Section 4).

The functions of the analysis of the demand

What has been proposed in the previous subsections of this section should have clarified the different functions that the analysis of the demand exerts within the process of the development of the client's request (Salvatore, 2016a).

The first function of the analysis of the demand lies in its enhancing the development of the request field by deconstructing the latter's premises of meaning. We define this function as *organizational* in the sense that it works to promote the conditions and regulatory devices of the client-psychologist relationship in order to optimize the intervention's capacity for effectiveness and utility. The qualitative and quantitative expansion of the big company's investment in the intervention reported previously is an example of the exercise of the organizational function of the analysis of the demand. It is worth recalling also that, as understood here, the term deconstructive is not synonymous with destructive. The premise of sense of the client system is both the constraint and the condition of development of the client's request. This means that the premise of sense must be enhanced and developed through the potential for innovative meanings they are capable of expressing rather than dismissed with the idea that they can be *tout court* replaced with another system of meaning that is more compatible with the psychologist's intervention project. Such a belief harkens back, *mutatis mutandis*, to the neocolonialist illusion of Western powers guaranteeing the viability of their own interests through the imposition of exogenous ruling classes in what had until recently been colonial possessions.

Analysis of the demand also has a *knowledge* function. As we have noted (Section 5.1; see also Figure 5.2), the demand reproduces the client's generalized system of meaning within the intersubjective field of the intervention. This means that the psychologist does not need to explore the client's living environment to detect their system of meaning. To abductively map it, it is sufficient to detect it in terms of how it is exercised – symbolically and performatively – within the relationship that the client establishes with the psychologist: in the way she/he presents herself/himself in the relationship, in the way of communicating, in the requests made, in the use of space and time, in the style as well as the content of the narratives, etc. This is clear at the level of the individual intervention since, as noted with regard to Mr. D.'s case, at that level, the demand can be conceptualized as an extended early form of the transferential-countertransferential dynamic, the analysis of which allows us to understand the generalized meaning that presides over the way the client interprets the experience. The knowledge function is, however, recognizably in operation also in the case of the request from the big company – the individualistic human resource model underlying the initial request is not a meaning exclusively concerned with how corporate management sees fit to proceed within the specific process of personnel recruitment – if it is so this is presumably because it is a general and pervasive organizational culture that informs the whole company life; an organizational culture that, by reason of operating in stable environments, represents organizational actors because of their characterological characteristics (Carli & Paniccia, 1999).

As to the latter consideration, it is worth noting that the possibility for the psychologist to use the demand as a source of knowledge is related to the fact that at a certain level of generalization (see Chapter 2), meanings tend to spread regardless of semantic, functional, space and time differences. This means that generalized meanings tend to be reproduced across contexts, regardless of circumstances, and spatial-temporal frameworks (for a similar idea, albeit based on a different theoretical framework, see Cole, 1996). It follows that the knowledge that the analysis of the demand produces relates only to meanings of a high level of generalization – self-other schemas, hyper-generalized meanings, and domain beliefs. The more specific the meaning is, the more it refers to circumscribed objects, and the less transferable it is since the more specific meanings are, the more they remain bound to the semantic and functional contexts within which they are produced. Thus, for example, if a client talking to the psychologist exhibits great wine expertise, this may suggest that there is a likelihood that they are also a good connoisseur of food and restaurants (a generalization within the domain related to good food), but not that they are also an expert in tennis or martial arts. In contrast, a client who exhibits their skills as trophies, we can assume, is exercising in the relationship with the psychologist a self-other schema (e.g., self as an object of admiration of the other) that they will tend to use in other domains of life as well.

It is also worth pointing out that the generalized meaning that substantiates the demand finds expression as much in the content as in the manner in which the request is made. Here the performative character of signs returns – meaning lies not only in the content of what is said but in the act of saying it. This is all the more relevant in the case of the analysis of the demand because the content of the request may largely depend on the institutional and functional canons that determine its conditions of expression. For example, turning to the psychotherapist inevitably tends to be configured according to a socio-institutional canon that assimilates the client's condition to that of the patient suffering from disease/illness. As a result, in psychotherapy, clients tend to report narratives of critical events and problematic experiences – and if they talk about positive aspects and events, they often do so to signal the change that has taken place. This leads to the conclusion that in addition to the content, the mode, the form of the client's saying and doing, their use of the space and time provide relevant information for the psychologist engaged in analyzing the demand (Salvatore et al., submitted). This suggests the possibility of introducing an additional rule – the *cretin rule*. The psychologist, like the cretin, when someone points to the moon, focuses on the finger.

Finally, analysis of the demand also fulfills an *intervention* function. As mentioned, analysis of the demand operates as a deconstructive vector aimed at elaborating innovative meanings capable of nurturing the development of the client. Such meanings, on the other hand, are not circumscribed within the perimeter of the request; they also inevitably inform the relationship between the client system and its world. The analysis of the demand then becomes a kind of hub of semiotic innovation, ready to release into the client's environment the resources of meaning produced therein. It comes in handy here again to refer to the analysis of the demand carried out in relation to the big company requesting the personnel selection intervention. The development of the request realized – a shift from personnel selection to organizational development – required and reflected the elaboration of a different organizational culture, characterized by the valorization of the relationship with the external environment as a driver of development. As already noted, the evolution of the client's organizational culture allowed the potential for the utility of the psychological intervention to be enhanced; at the same time, the progressive expression of this potential further nurtured the development of the client, thus the organizational culture at its foundation, constituting itself from this point of view as a further vector of change.

It is also useful here to recall a methodological criterion. The psychologist is called upon to calibrate the focus of analysis of the demand to the level of meaning relevant to the intervention. In fact, as we have already observed, meanings of different levels of generalization are all present at the same time. Or rather, the meaning is only one; what varies are the levels to which it can be ascribed. It is therefore up to the psychologist to choose the appropriate level because of the semiotic resources the intervention seeks to develop. For example, the request of the large company can, in principle, also be interpreted in terms of maximum generalization – that is to say, at the level of the affective self-other schema. The psychoanalytically oriented psychosociological tradition offers many examples of such interpretations (e.g., Carli & Paniccia, 1981). Yet, the analysis of the demand associated with this request focused appropriately on the level of meaning related to what we have termed domain beliefs – namely, the organizational culture underlying the way the company makes sense of its environment and designs/pursues its projects. This is because it is at this level of meaning that it is useful for the client system to develop the ability to recognize its own premises of sense and thus define innovative ways of engaging with its reality. In contrast, where, as in the case of individual intervention, the psychologist's action concerns taking charge of the relationship between the client and their world as a whole, it then becomes useful to identify the level of meaning on which to anchor the analysis as the self-other schema.

6 Result and value of the intervention. Output and outcome

The previous section highlights how the request, thus the demand that under-lies it, impacts intervention not only in defining the conditions and constraints within which the psychologist's action can be exercised but also in qualifying the value of its outcome. We devote this section to the second aspect.

End and objective

Intervention is a purposeful, goal-oriented, competent action. The request is also a purposive action – the psychologist is believed to serve to achieve some result. However, the logical architecture underlying the two types of action is different to a significant degree. It is, therefore, appropriate to explore this dif-ference in depth so as to identify the form of their possible relationship. In this perspective, it is useful to refer to the distinction proposed by Carli between the *end* and the *objective* of the intervention (Carli, 1987b).

The *end* is a perspective of social desirability, defined in terms of values. Peace, freedom, universal brotherhood, and justice are examples of an end – beliefs about what is good and worth pursuing that, like the North Star, indi-cate the direction in which to aim. Ends are an asymptotic goal in the sense that they do not denote specific empirical qualities of reality; they are abstract and generalized concepts (field signs, cf. Valsiner, 2014), to which, therefore, no state of the world is able to correspond – for example, what human reality corresponds to the realization of justice? Moreover, precisely because of their abstract nature, ends are inherently polysemous. The meaning of terms such as peace, justice, and freedom depends on the web of meanings of which these signs are part. What is the pursuit of an end for one person is the negation of it for someone else. History is a collection of shenanigans produced by the way people have believed they were pursuing the noblest and highest ends. As we are writing, the tanks of a foreign power are driving through a sovereign country, sowing death and destruction for the purpose of "securing peace." In sum, ends give meaning and motivate action as they qualify it as a way to pursue a socially desirable goal – striving for justice, bringing peace to the world, promoting the common good, etc.

The *objective*, on the other hand, is the representation of the expected output of a competent action – the state of reality that, because of contextual conditions, a given network of operations is expected to reach/determine. This definition implies five aspects that deserve to be highlighted. First, as defined, the objective is a concept that corresponds to a state of reality, thus empirically qualifiable and representable. Peace is an end; a peace treaty is an objective. Second, the goal is necessarily contingent; that is, it depends on contextual conditions. In other words, the possible output of any action varies as a function of the available resources (temporal, symbolic, economic, etc.). The surgeon operating in a field hospital in a war zone does not set himself the same objectives as the surgeon performing the same operation at the Massachusetts General Hospital in Boston. Third, as a corollary to the previous point, the objective is necessarily circumscribed – pursuing one objective implies choosing not to pursue another. Fourth, the objective implies an inference of a Bayesian nature – it represents the *expected* output of the action, prefigured because of a given a priori knowledge of the relationship between the action itself and its possible impact. Finally, the objective defines a normative linkage between the action and its output: the action is expected to achieve its pursued objective; if this does not happen, it is inferred that an error has occurred and that the action has met with failure. The normativity of the objective is an essential condition both for regulating the action – if the objective were not binding, one could not keep the action-oriented to it – and, more generally, for learning – one learns to the extent that one can correct an error, but without normativity, there would be no error, any output would be fine. It deserves to be noted that the normative quality of the goal is not contradictory to its contingent and Bayesian nature. On the contrary, such a quality is possible precisely because of these characteristics – the tie between action and its output is sustainable insofar as it is defined by reason of the context and in probabilistic terms. In other words, the action prescriptively assumes as its output a given probability distribution; the one judged appropriate to the contextual conditions by the knowledge on which the action is based.

The relationship between end and objective is hermeneutic, not functional. The end provides the frame of meaning within which the objective is defined. This definition consists of the formulation of a state of reality consistent with the end, thus representable as a local and contingent way of moving in the direction of the end. Eliminating educational poverty is an end; reducing by x% the rate of school dropout in a given area is an objective that – in that given context and with the resources available, given the intervention models available and the studies related to their impact – represents the optimal way to move in the direction indicated by the end. The interpretation of the end and its use to formulate the objective implies thus the convergence of two references. On the one hand, the understanding of the socio-institutional value expressed by the end: as noted, the objective makes sense to the extent that it remains consistent with the end. On the other, the functional constraints (context, resources, operational models) define the possibilities of professional action to achieve a given output.

There is a rather widespread tendency in psychology to treat ends as if they were objectives. Consider, in this sense, how widespread within psychological discourse are representations of the profession as an action aimed at promoting well-being, health, and resilience. Such concepts do not denote empirically definable states of reality, but rather – not unlike peace, justice, and freedom – socially desirable values toward which to strive (for a discussion of this in relation to the use in psychology of the concept of health, see Salvatore, 2021b). This tendency reflects a more general socio-institutional mechanism: given their value-driven weight, ends promote the consensus and social legitimacy of the practices associated with them. On ends, we all agree – who can say they are opposed to peace, justice, and freedom? Those who represent themselves as committed to pursuing them can aspire to enjoy, through a kind of metonymic contagion, the social favor they produce. Because of this mechanism, professional action assumes legitimacy by the very fact that it is performed, regardless of the result it produces. Consider, as an example of this mechanism, the disproportion that exists between the centrality that psychologists attribute to primary prevention interventions and the limited availability of operational models aimed at implementing such interventions and, even more so, of studies that assess their impacts.

Confusing ends and objectives can further the legitimization of the professional function, especially from a short- to medium-term perspective. However, professional action needs to keep the two terms distinct and related. Ends mediate the relationship with society. It thus operates as a linkage between the professional system and society. Indeed, the request for action tends to be inevitably shaped by the ends. This is so because the definition of pursuable objective, as noted above, requires techno-scientific competencies that are held by the psychologist, not by the client system. This is always true – one goes to the practitioner to feel well, one buys a cell phone to feel in touch with the world, one chooses the electric car to make a contribution to the survival of the planet, etc. One only has to take a quick look at the advertising messages that bombard us to realize how the client's request is fueled by the symbolic value of the product/service, that is, by its ability to anchor itself to a socially valued end. On the other hand, for those responsible for professional action, taking the end as if it were the objective to be accomplished is equivalent to proposing to empty the ocean with a spoon. As noted, the end is an asymptotic, polysemic perspective, void of empirical content – anything performed in its name, while reproducing it as a value, is inevitably doomed to failure when understood as a way to achieve a factual state. In short, treating ends as a goal is like trying to reach the horizon. A professional action that does not translate the ends mobilizing the request into a realistically achievable objective will feed on social legitimacy but at the cost of a structural weakening of the ability to represent its actual impact, and thus to regulate itself, learn from experience, and develop – in short, to consolidate its identity as a socio-technical system aimed at generating utility for clients and society.

The considerations offered in different parts of this book should have highlighted the reasons why it is more complicated for psychology than for other professions to distinguish and connect ends and objectives. On the one hand, psychological theories of change, especially when one moves to scales other than individual and micro-social, have limited explanatory power due both to their domain-specific focus and to their difficulty in conceptualizing the mechanisms that mediate the relationship between operations and outputs (see Chapter 1). On the other hand, the symbolic and institutional weakness of psychology makes it less easy for the client to give up the ends that fuel its request. The patient to whom the practitioner has communicated that it will be impossible to find a cure but only to limit the course of the illness may seek other opinions but, in the end, will tend to accept the objective proposed by the expert. This happens less easily in the case of psychology: not infrequently, the request addressed to the psychologist is fueled by ends so close to the client's self-identity vision that it is difficult for the client to distance themselves from it.

Objective and impact

From the discussion presented in the previous section, it follows that the objective is the immediate output of the action. Immediate, not in the temporal sense, but in the sense of non-mediated by contextual conditions – i.e., the outcome is not influenced by circumstances external to the intervention. As we have pointed out, this is because the contextual conditions are incorporated upstream in the local and contingent definition of the objective. Thus, the logical structure of the objective takes on the following pattern: (1) due to context conditions C, (2) action A, (3) will determine with probability p, (4) the output O.

If C, then A -> $p_{(O)}$

The immediateness of the objective is an essential condition. Only under this condition, in fact, can the psychological intervention sustain the normative link between action and the result pursued, thus using the latter to regulate the action and, at the same time, to assume responsibility for the result with the client system.

It follows that it is necessary to distinguish the *objective* of the intervention from its *impact*, where with the latter term, we refer to the effects that the output produces because of and within the context. The distinction at stake here is epistemic, not ontological: a given change is considered an objective if and only if the psychologist, on the basis of a theory of change, can consider it the direct, immediately derivable output of the intervention. Conversely, if such a change involves the action of additional elements exogenous to the intervention, then it deserves to be considered an impact. The distinction, moreover, is not absolute but contingent – it depends on the theory of change and the boundaries of the intervention – that is, on the one hand, on what connections the scientific knowledge underlying the intervention establishes between the professional action and its immediate consequences, and on the other hand, on the aspects of the relationship with the client over which the intervention extends its action. In other words, this means that what is to be considered impact in a given intervention can be conceived of as objective in a different intervention situation.

The distinction between objective and impact is not specific to psychology. The objective of medical therapy is to eradicate the virus and bring the organism back within physiological parameters of functioning, while allowing the sick person to return to work is one of the possible impacts. The programmer's objective is the software they propose to design, while the profit of the company that produces it is one of the possible impacts. In psychology, however, the distinction is more complicated because of the lack of clarity about what should be considered internal and what should be considered external to the black box (see Chapter 3). Often, objectives are defined in terms of behaviors: of reducing socially undesirable conduct – for example, think of interventions focused on addictions, risk behaviors, school dropouts, cyberbullying, and gender-based violence – or of promoting positively connoted ways of acting – think of interventions aimed at promoting more rewarding relational modes, healthy lifestyles, civic participation, or pro-environment choices. In our view, this way of representing the purpose of the intervention is appropriate to the extent that it is understood as relating to impact; it instead becomes critical when it is treated as relating to an objective. This is, for a fundamental reason, discussed earlier (see Chapters 1 and 2): the lack of an invariant link between the psychological dynamic – i.e., sensemaking – and the way it is instantiated at the level of observable behavior. Any pattern of sensemaking can feed into a plurality of behavioral modes and, conversely, the same behavior can be an expression of a plurality of patterns of signification. This is not to say that there is no nexus between meaning and behavior. This nexus, however, is locally defined by reason of the network of meanings involved. For example, idealization of the adult figure (pattern of meaning) may lead some students, because of the role played by a plurality of contextual and individual factors, to invest in their relationship with the teacher and thus in their schoolwork (behavior) and others to experience that relationship as challenging to the point of feeling it necessary to abandon it (opposite behavior). Again, research has shown that behavior opposed to anti-COVID vaccination is fueled by different beliefs and contextual interpretations, which are also very different from each other – for some, the refusal of vaccination is an expression of radical distrust in institutions; for others, a critique of the commodification of health care resources, and for still others an act of defense against an attempt at conspiratorial manipulation perpetrated by strong powers (Graffigna, 2021).

How, then, to define the objective of intervention?

The theory of change discussed in Chapter 3 provides a way to answer this question. Intervention is ultimately a device for activating a process of semiotic change. From this point of view, it is configured as a *methodological exercise* which does not pursue specific states of reality. In other words, it is not defined as a transition from state A to state B but as a way of activating a development trajectory of the client dynamic of sensemaking (Carli, 1987b). Depending on the circumstances of intervention, this trajectory will be prefigured in terms of a semiotic change of type 1, 2, or 3, or their combination (see Chapter 3).

One final clarification before concluding this section. The methodological nature of the goal is not inconsistent with the fact that the intervention possesses an inherent normative valence: professional action pursues a change that is assumed to correspond to the achievement of a state of increased desirability. The methodological nature and normative valence of the intervention are not contradictory, however, as the latter concerns the impact, not the objective. The impact is normatively definable in that its value is defined because of the client's intended end. In other words, the intervention activates a process (methodological objective) whose meaning/consequence for the client (impact) can be represented normatively by the client, i.e., in terms of how much the professional action has fostered the determination of a desirable state of affairs.

The dimensions of the psychologist's responsibility

In the previous section, we put forward the argument that the objective of the intervention is limited to the immediate output of the action to be distinguished from the impact. Yet, the responsibility that the psychologist takes for the objective – which we will refer to in what follows as *technical responsibility* – is not the only thing for which the professional must account. Given its methodological nature, the output of the intervention – the process of semiotic change triggered by the professional action – taken in itself has no content, either functional or social. It takes on content always, and only because of its context, that is to say, because of and in terms of its impact. This leads to the recognition that intervention must be parameterized because of two levels of impact, corresponding to two dimensions of responsibility, the *functional* and the *political*.

By *functional responsibility*, we mean the recognition of the fact that at the moment they accept the client's request, the psychologist, in fact, recognizes that the objective they are going to pursue is not the purpose of the intervention but the means by which the client intends to obtain a utility. In short, functional responsibility is the psychologist's recognition that the output of the intervention must be at the service of – i.e., it must be functional for – a utility and that it finds meaning and value in that.

It should be noted that the relationship between the objective and its utility cannot be drawn in linear terms. Utility does not increase steadily as the technical quality of the output increases. In fact, while it is true that a low level of output's technical quality results in an equally low utility – for example, ineffective psychotherapy (low technical quality of the output) does not generate adaptive potential for the patient (low utility) – it is equally true that an output may be of inappropriate utility by excess – for example, a psychodiagnostic assessment that collects data on aspects that are not strictly necessary produces an extremely rich evaluative picture (high technical quality of the output) that nevertheless harms rather than benefits the client (low utility) – for example, in terms of cost and waiting time.

This raises a practical and conceptual problem of no small magnitude. As noted, the objective is the expected output as an immediate consequence of the psychologist's competent action. Consequently, the psychologist can take (technical) responsibility for the output – it will mean the success of the intervention if it is achieved or failure the other way around. In other words, once defined in form and content, because of contextual conditions, the objective constitutes a "promise" that the psychologist undertakes to keep. By contrast, the utility of the output (i.e., its impact) depends on the interaction between the output, the client's project grounding its use/valorization, and the contextual conditions that mediate such use and its consequences. Hence, the psychologist cannot take direct responsibility for a variable (utility) whose values reflect the client's sphere of autonomy and its context. How, then, can the psychologist adopt the criterion of functional responsibility as a parameter for regulating their professional action?

Our answer to this question is based on the distinction between *endogenous* and *exogenous* regulation of functional responsibility. The two forms of regulation can be considered the extremes of a continuum – every intervention, in fact, is characterized by a mix of these two modalities.

Endogenous regulation is based on the development of clients, on making them more capable (see Section 3), that is, the promotion of the competence of the client system to use the output of the intervention. We call this form of regulation of functional responsibility endogenous in that it is carried out from within the intervention, as its function of promoting the quality of the client's project of using the output, the latter being understood as part of its demand. Endogenous regulation can be represented by the following formula:

$$U = f(O, C)$$

Where U stands for Usefulness, O for Output, and C for Competence of Use.

In summary, endogenous regulation consists of the optimization of the utility of the intervention's impact through the enhancement of the two terms on the right-hand side of the formula: the greater the optimization of the output with respect to the client's project and the greater the client's competence to use that output, the greater the utility to the client from the intervention.

Incidentally, the endogenous regulation of functional responsibility recalls in the field of psychological intervention the logic of service management (Norman, 1986). Services are a special category of economic activity, characterized, among other things, by the fact that in them, it is not possible to distinguish between the moment of delivery and the moment of fruition – service is inherently relational: it takes place in the interaction between provider and user. Consequently, the value of a service depends on how the output of the service is interpreted by the client, where this interpretation is realized commensurately with the service production. A work of art, a dinner at a restaurant, and a stay in a hotel are examples of activities whose value is not intrinsic to the output but is determined by the experience that the user has of it, thus by the client's project of use. From this point of view, endogenous regulation implies conceiving psychological intervention in terms of service: the psychologist does not circumscribe their responsibility to the technical dimension of the immediate output produced but assumes as anchorage the utility/value that the output generates in the interaction with the client system.

Exogenous regulation operates where the competence of use is not developable. In this case, the relationship between output and impact relies on the mediation of the socio-institutional context. That is, it is assumed that given the relevant conditions of the sociocultural and institutional environment – e.g., value system, social practice patterns, distribution of social capital – a given outcome will be associated with a given probabilistic distribution of utility values. Such an assumption may be based, as is often the case, on a recognition of the regularities that are present within the cultural contexts of reference, thus keeping to the plane of practical knowledge that presides over the understanding of these contexts. It can, on the other hand, be validated through ad hoc studies – as has happened, for example, in the field of verifying the effects of psychotherapies, where the analysis of clinical effectiveness has, in several cases, been supplemented by the estimation of the impact of clinical changes on patients' capacities for social adaptation and life development. Endogenous adjustment can be represented by the following formula:

$$U = f(O, E)$$

Where U stands for Utility, O for Output, and E for sociocultural environment.

For example, a recent study (Madeo et al., 2021) has shown that identification with more complex meanings in the cultural context of Western societies results in more civic-oriented behavior. From this, it can be deduced that given the contextual conditions (E), increased complexity of sensemaking (O) translates into utility – obviously to the extent that the growth of civicness is seen as such.

Political responsibility is about recognizing the consequences – social, institutional, economic, and ecological – of the intervention's impact on beneficiaries and stakeholders. The smaller the involvement of these actors in the intervention, the greater the political responsibility for the intervention. We use the political attribute here as Di Maria (2005, 2021) proposes it, namely, as a form of social life aimed at building the common good. We prefer to speak of political rather than ethical responsibility since, in the meaning with which we use the former term, it seems to us to be more inclusive – capable of taking into account the axiological dimension, as well as fundamental ideas about ways of organizing social, institutional and economic relations. Let us give a few examples. A few years ago, we learned of American psychologists who, in their role as advisors of the CIA, had devised a series of interrogation techniques operating as real torture used to obtain information needed to identify those responsible for the attack on the Twin Towers and protect the United States from further terrorist attacks. Consider, again, the not infrequent cases of requests that involve triangulation/manipulation with beneficiaries positioned in positions of power asymmetry – e.g., requests for training programs designed as ways to "normalize" employees, parents requesting the psychologist's intervention because of unrealistic and self-referenced expectations about what is good for their offspring. In cases like those, the client's utility project inevitably conflicts with the interests and rights of third parties and challenges the psychologist on the political (as understood here) level, even before the technical one.

Political responsibility raises two orders of questions: how to map such conflict? what responsibility does the psychologist assume with respect to it?

With regard to the first question, it must first be acknowledged that it is not possible to define an absolute normative standpoint on the basis of which to establish a dividing line between universally lawful and actionable client utilities such that they can, therefore, be supported/assimilated by the psychologist, and utilities, on the other hand, that contrast with the obligations arising from the psychologist's political responsibility. Rarely can the client's utility projects be blatantly and unambiguously politically unacceptable. On this point, let us return to the case of the psychologists advising the CIA torturers. One of them publicly vindicated his work, stating during a public hearing that he would do it all over again because he considered it his moral duty to protect his countrymen and that this duty was more relevant to the principle of not harming the alleged terrorists who were the victims of the interrogators since the latter had voluntarily decided to attack the American people. Our thesis is that the only way to untangle the skein of viewpoints involved – without succumbing to the opposing temptation to deny the complexity of the perspectives involved and to embrace a form of relativism with a postmodernist flavor – is to assume a *negative, pluralist* logic of evaluation. This means that the psychologist's political responsibility is expressed as an unwillingness to take on the components of the client's request that contrast with the constraints of political responsibility. In other words, the psychologist welcomes the request unless there is a well-founded possibility that her/ his intervention will produce an impact assessable as a politically illegitimate violation of third-party interests and rights. This assessment emerges from the combination of three points of view: 1) the scientific-professional community (as organized by the institutional arrangements that regulate its functioning, (e.g., professional associations, code of ethics); 2) the institutional framework of the rule of law; and 3) the professional's sense of citizenship and value system. It is enough for just one of these three points of view to lead to an assessment of the impact of the intervention as politically illegitimate in order to bind the psychologist to the responsibility of making themselves unavailable to take on the client's request.

Note

1 www.fabriziodeandre.it/faber/wp-content/uploads/2019/07/Il-testamento-di-Tito_eng-version.pdf; www.youtube.com/watch?v=16LCnH1YjCY

6

LEVELS OF THE INTERVENTION

This concluding chapter is devoted to presenting some conceptual frameworks and case examples of the ways in which the GTPI presented in the previous chapters enable the development of interpretative models of phenomena and strategies/formats of intervention on them. Our intention is not to define an exhaustive map of the potential uses of GTPI. Rather, we are interested in showing how referring to the general idea of psychology as a science of sense-making offers a way of conceiving the psychological function in a unified way in relation to a wide range of different phenomena in a plurality of domains and scales of observation, without this entailing a loss of the ability to calibrate the intervention because of the specificity of the problem activating it. We considered it useful to select cases from among those in which the authors of this book were directly involved. This is to give a biographical sign of how reference to a general theory of psychological intervention allows individual practitioners to operate on a wide and transversal range of fields of action, problems, and forms of commissioning.

The chapter is divided into three parts, each referring to a phenomenal level. The first section concerns the individual and interpersonal relationship level and focuses on the reading of psychopathology and psychotherapy in terms of sensemaking. The second section presents two intervention cases that address issues on the meso-social level. In both cases, the psychological intervention focuses on the semiotic resources and is configured as a strategy aimed at enhancing them. The third section discusses two methodological criteria – symbolic policy and intermediate processes – that represent the implications of GTPI at the macro-social level.

DOI: 10.4324/9781003449362-7

1 Individual and interpersonal level

Psychopathology and dimensionality of affective signification

As we have noted (in particular, Chapters 2 and 3), according to the psycho-semiotic theory of mind, subjective experience consists of the components of the intersubjective field made relevant by generalized affective meanings (the ground; see Chapter 2, Section 2). This means that what the person feels, thinks, and how they act is inscribed within and constrained by these components, by the variability within them. For example, imagine an individual who experiences the world in terms of the affective ground of pleasantness/unpleasantness; for such an individual, the experience of the world is substantiated by the intersubjective scenario of swinging between a state of satisfaction and one of dissatisfaction. Consequently, feelings, beliefs, decisions, expectations, predictions, and actions – that is, the person's subjective, interpersonal, and socio-institutional life – will move within the horizon of sense defined by this variation in the affective ground.

It follows that psychopathology can be conceived as reflecting the limited dimensionality of the affective ground, i.e., the subject's tendency to constitute the contents of experience in terms of pertinentizing a limited number of components of the intersubjective field. As a result of this, the subject remains blind to many environmental components of variation that are important in governing trajectories of adaptation and, more generally, in making life meaningful (Venuleo et al., 2020). If you will, psychopathology is like color blindness, which makes the person unable to recognize a variety of colors, preventing them from both gathering significant information from the environment (e.g., traffic light color) and enjoying the hues of the sunset.

Considering psychopathology in terms of the low dimensionality of the affective ground is consistent with the idea that clinical psychological phenomena are to be interpreted in terms of the rigidity of the psychic apparatus. Concepts such as the rigidity of internal operating models, low flexibility of defense mechanisms, the repetitiveness of maladaptive interpersonal patterns, and saturated group matrix are all indicative of this general idea. The psycho-semiotic notion of dimensionality offers an explanation of the mechanism underlying rigidity, modeling it on the computational level as a function of the low dimensionality of the affective ground. Just as a sprinter can walk while a person not dedicated to competitive athletics is unable to run the 100 meters in under ten seconds, similarly, a high dimensional affective ground can be reduced when this is appropriate to the circumstances (e.g., when the person goes to the stadium), while the opposite is not possible. Thus, a subject characterized by low-dimensional affective semiosis can only make sense of the world in the terms, and within the constraints, of a system of meaning unable to capture the nuances of meaning that substantiate the quality of life.

M. is a 22-year-old woman suffering from anxiety and emotional instability. She decided to seek psychotherapy because two years after separation from her partner, she continues to suffer from it – she does not wish to return to him but cannot imagine him engaged in a relationship with someone other than herself. An only child, she lives with her mother, who is separated from her husband and who is totally devoted to her daughter. During her teenage years, M. was involved in theatre, achieving excellent results and systematically becoming the teacher's favorite. She has always had many friends who appreciate her for her cheerful nature and helpfulness. In discussions, she has the first and last word, convinced that her own view of how things should be is the right one. No feelings or attitudes of arrogance are associated with this basic conviction, and her friends, in most circumstances, show that they share it. About a year after starting psychotherapy, she manifested some potentially alarming physical symptoms. This triggered a long course of analysis and clinical consultations, which fostered intense hypochondriac concerns, only marginally alleviated by the systematic reassuring outcomes of assessments. As the psychotherapeutic work allowed her to understand, what fueled her strong belief that she was terminally ill was not the clinical data but the feeling that the doctors did not accept her request to be taken care of. Similarly, what calmed M. was not the reassuring results of the examinations but the fact that she had met a doctor who had welcomed her need to be taken in charge.

In sum, M. seems to shape experience in terms of being/not being the target of the object's totalizing love. Because of this affective ground, M. alternates between a state of contentment and stability and an opposite state of anxiety and apathy. Her contentment reflects a world that allows itself to be interpreted affectively as ready to love her exclusively and totally. For example, the way her mother, teachers, and her understanding doctor appreciate her are experienced by M. as putting her at the center of their minds and using her feelings and reactions as criteria for regulating their own internal states and actions. In the opposite state of anxiety and apathy, the object (ex-boyfriend, reluctant doctors) is experienced as unresponsive to her request to be loved. In terms of the dimensional view of psychopathology discussed previously, these two juxtaposed intersubjective fields can be modeled as a ground, consisting of two dimensions of bimodal affective meaning: |good/bad| and |powerful/powerless|. The combination of the |good and powerful| polarities maps the self-perception that M. experiences when she feels she is filled by the object's love; |bad and powerless| substantiates the opposite connotation of being rejected by the object.

M.'s vicissitudes related to clinical ascertainment exemplify how such a low-dimensional model can limit the detection of resources (meanings, relations, institutional devices) available in the environment and, in so doing, hinder the elaboration of forms of relationship with it that are useful to the subject. For instance, given the limited dimensionality of meaning underlying the way M. maps the intersubjective field, her relationship with clinicians cannot but focus on the clinician's attitude toward her and what this attitude tells about her ability to be loved. As a result, the clinical data regarding her health – ultimately: the reality function of that field of action – end up being backgrounded.

It would be beyond the scope of this paper to delve into the question of the causes of low-dimensional ground. Here, we will simply say that it is plausible to assume that the dimensionality of the affective ground emerges from the way early relational experiences are processed (refer in this regard to Salvatore, De Luca Picione et al., 2022). Overly simplified or overly complex (i.e., chaotic) forms of early self-world relations make the development of the dimensionality of affective ground unnecessary (for an initial empirical validation of this hypothesis, based on a simulation design, see Kleinbub et al., 2021; Antonucci et al., 2022). From this point of view, the development of the dimensionality of the affective ground can be conceptualized in analogy with language acquisition: the less the world requires the subject to have a certain syntactic or semantic competence in order to linguistically regulate the relationship with it, the less the subject will be driven to develop this competence, thus to internalize it as an organizer of future linguistic activity.

It should be pointed out that the view of psychopathology as a function of the dimensionality of affective semiosis is consistent with and provides an explanatory framework to the line of thought that has been developing in recent years, which emphasizes the unitary character of psychopathology. According to this approach, the many forms that mental illness takes are manifestations of a single underlying psychopathological process. This thesis has found convincing empirical support – research has indeed been able to show that clinical syndromes generally thought to be independent share a considerable portion of covariation – the so-called *p-factor* (Caspi et al., 2014). However, there has yet to be found an agreement on the clinical interpretation of the p-factor and, more importantly, on how it operates. The dimensional model outlined previously offers one possible way to address this issue (Venuleo et al., 2020).

Psychotherapeutic process as an intersubjective field

Psycho-semiotic theory leads to the conception of the psychotherapeutic process as an *intersubjective field* (Salvatore & Gennaro, 2015). As understood here, the intersubjective field is the context of affective meanings emerging from the interaction of the structural (e.g., treatment conditions, duration) and dynamic (e.g., therapeutic interventions, experiences, elaborative styles, defense mechanisms, transferential and counter-transferential dynamics, adopted narratives, thematic content, discursive forms) elements that characterize the *here and now* of the clinical exchange. The intersubjective field is constantly fed and reproduced over time by the communicative acts (and corresponding intrapsychic configurations) that substantiate the clinical exchange.

At the same time, recursively, the intersubjective field shapes the form of these communication processes and their interpretation. In other words, the intersubjective field defines the conditions and constraints under which the elements of the therapeutic process interact with each other and, in so doing, generate clinical impact. This means that the interwoven interpretations of the exchange that bind patient and therapist are not realized as products of isolated minds but take shape because of the intersubjective field that comes into being between the participant to the exchange. The conceptualization of the psychotherapeutic process in terms of the intersubjective field thus implies the idea that the clinical exchange operates as a regulator of the participants' mental processes (Rocco et al., 2017; Salvatore et al., 2010).

A description of the micro-dynamic of the intersubjective field underlying the therapeutic process is offered by the *Two Stage Semiotic Model* (TSSM) (Gennaro et al., 2011; Salvatore et al., 2010). Underlying the TSSM is the idea of the clinical exchange as an intersubjective process of co-construction of meaning aimed at changing the affective and cognitive mode in which the patient makes sense of the experience. Patients come to psychotherapy with a tendentially rigid system of superordinate generalized meanings (affective self-other schemas, metacognitive modes, conceptions of the world, relational strategies, and so on) that operate as premises of sense that regulate how experience is interpreted. These premises represent both the source of the criticality that leads the patient to seek intervention and the foundation/constraint of valorizing the relationship with the therapist. Symptoms, intrapsychic, and relational conflicts can be conceived as the way in which such superordinate meanings are expressed and reproduced (Bucci, 1997). This leads to the conclusion that the premises of sense that substantiate the patient's system of meaning are the motive, the object, the goal, and the mediator of the psychotherapeutic intervention.

The TSSM describes the process of meaning co-construction as a cyclical dynamic fueled by the alternation of two phases. More specifically, the model maintains that a clinically effective psychotherapeutic process is characterized by the alternation between a phase in which a deconstructive form of sensemaking prevails (deconstructive stage) and another in which the clinical exchange fuels the patient's activity of exploration and creation of new meanings (constructive stage). In the initial moments of treatment, the clinical dialogue exposes the patient to a different system of meaning, the one conveyed by the therapeutic setting and the associated vectors activated by the psychotherapist (see Chapter 4). This difference operates as a potential source of constraint on the patient's meaning system. Thanks to the constraining function exerted by the setting, the clinical exchange may not allow itself to be saturated by the patient's own way of interpreting the relationship with the therapist, therefore reproducing within it the critical elements (e.g., way of thinking, feelings, behaviors, and attitudes) that the clinical exchange is called upon to address. For example, a paranoid patient who considers everyone eager to attack and destroy him will have little chance of benefiting from psychotherapy if he assimilates the therapist to his own paranoid schema and thus feels that the latter aims to hurt him. This first phase is thus basically a deconstructive process in which the therapeutic dialogue functions as an external constraint on the regulatory activity of the patient's problematic superordinate meanings. The weakening of the patient's superordinate critical meaning paves the way for the second phase of psychotherapy, characterized by the patient's elaboration of new meanings. In the second phase, the patient-therapist dialogue allows the emergence of new superordinate meanings, which supplement and modify the previous system of premises. Once the meanings emerge, they are consolidated, creating the conditions for a new deconstructive phase, and so on, according to a continuous two-phase dynamic.

2 Meso-social level

A prevention strategy for adolescents[1]

This section illustrates the model of intervention targeting adolescents elaborated in the context of a consultation for an agency engaged in psychological interventions aimed at promoting well-being and counteracting forms of distress in adolescents and young adults. Over the previous years, the agency had built an effective workshop format, used as a clinical intervention device aimed at adolescents experiencing psychological and social problems. The client was interested in developing this format further to expand its function from the already established one of secondary prevention to that of primary prevention. This meant redesigning the workshop in order to make it consistent with the two main characteristics of primary prevention interventions: 1) *systemic extension* – i.e., primary prevention has the population at large as its target, rather than relatively large groups of users identified due to a risk factor; and 2) *developmental function* – i.e., primary prevention interventions are aimed at enhancing/developing conditions of normality, rather than counteracting conditions of risk and/or overcoming criticality.

With guidance, support, and advisors, the agency's team, composed of psychologists and other professionals involved in conducting workshops, made a systematic analysis of the workshop format used up to that time. On this basis, an *extended workshop model* (hereafter: EWM) was developed, designed to pursue primary prevention goals. In what follows, we outline the essential features of the EWM as the advisors systematized it.

The purpose of the EWM is defined from a psycho-semiotic perspective. The EWM aims to contribute to the *development of semiotic resources that are accessible to the youth population*. More specifically, the primary prevention goal of the EWM is the promotion of innovative cultural models (*semiotic capital,* see Section 4) that substantiate young people's ability to mentalize context, thus the socio-cognitive competencies (beliefs, temporality, images of otherness) required to regulate the transition into the adult world. This definition is based on the theoretical assumption that the cognitive processes that nurture/constrain the behavioral forms of adaptation and transition to the adult world are ultimately the intrapsychic precipitate of the semiotic resources present within the cultural milieu in which subjects are immersed (see Chapter 2).

Consistently with its purpose, the EWM defines its target client on two levels, distinguishing between *proximal* and *distal* users. Primary prevention interventions cannot, for obvious reasons of feasibility, extend directly over the entire target client (i.e., the entire youth population of the area). Consequently, the users participating in the workshops (proximal clients) should be considered instrumentally as a vector for multiplying/propagating the innovative meanings generated locally (i.e., in the workshops) for the benefit of the entire target population (distal users).

The distinction between the two planes of target/impact (proximal/distal) can be made because of the semiotic-cultural reformulation of the EWM purpose. Indeed, semiotic resources, unlike individual cognitive skills/processes, are by definition endowed with the capacity for diffusion within the population. From this point of view, the EWM integrates two levels of action: 1) the use of laboratories as incubators of innovative cultural models; and 2) the provision of conditions for the diffusion of such models within the meso-social fabric of the active youth population of the area.

The two levels of action are pursued through the systematic and intensified exercise of the fundamental methodological principle of the performativity of the intervention setting. In short, this principle asserts that the development and dissemination of meanings – particularly the level of affective meanings that substantiate the semiotic capital – do not come about through consensual agreement or declarative endorsement of values; rather, semiotic resources are implicitly shaped and propagated through being embedded in social practices (see Chapter 2). Moreover, the more these social practices are relevant to the target's identity, the easier it is to identify with them.

This gives rise, on the methodological level, to the principle that to promote innovative meanings, it is necessary to design and implement social practices that have such meanings at their foundation; social practices, moreover, that are identity-relevant for the subjects involved, i.e., that have a significant role in defining the subjective, existential landscape of these subjects.

The EWM derives from the principle of the performativity of meaning of three setting parameters:

1. semiotic mediation (usability);
2. role hybridization (prosumers);
3. systemic integration (adoptability).

Semiotic mediation. The workshop activity is aimed at the realization of outputs endowed with value. In other words, the products created by the adolescents are not mere pretexts used to enable the workshop to operate as a context for socialization. The non-pretextual nature of the workshop products is enhanced through the choice of outputs with a high value of *interpretive usability* – not merely artifacts (e.g., ashtrays, canvas bags), but artifacts that can serve as resources that generate the sense and representability of the experience, for proximal, distal users and stakeholders – e.g., musical texts, artistic works, radio programs, photographs. In other words, the EWM accentuates the *semiotic nature* of the workshop outputs. This is done by designing and pursuing the output in modes that increase not only their *ecological validity* – that is, artifacts endowed with value within the adult world – but also their *epistemic validity* – that is, artifacts capable of mapping domains of meaning, thus generating innovative forms of representability of contexts.

It is worth highlighting that this choice of intensifying the interpretive value of products does not have a merely motivational purpose. It constitutes an exercise in performativity aimed at determining a form of social practice within which the young participants in the workshop can experience themselves as producers of signs not only capable of being received by the adult world but also, above all, capable in some way of re-signifying it.

Role hybridization. Proximal users (youth participants in the workshops) are required to assume a twofold role: in addition to the obvious position of users of the activities and resources of the workshop, they are encouraged (through specific *affordances* provided by the setting) to assume functions of co-management of the workshop's process of production. This is the prosumer (*producer-consumer*) model inherent to the logic of service (Norman, 1986), revisited according to the goals of the psychological intervention. The position of prosumer implies a system of regulation of the workgroup based on the recognition of its organizational context of its constraints: as a co-participant in the process of production and its regulation, the workshop participants find themselves, in fact, immersed in a reality that induces them to take charge of the overall functioning of the work group. In other words, in addition to playing, the workshop participant is called on to be involved in game maintenance. This fosters the development of skills in regulating one's own behavior, recognizing the other's standpoint, and negotiating with it.

Systemic integration. The greater the processes and products of the workshops are interconnected with the institutional contexts that structure and regulate the daily lives of the adolescents involved, the more they can operate as generative vectors of meaning. From this perspective, a continuum of the systemic integration of workshops can be outlined: the *low-integration level* is related to the linkage mediated exclusively by the artifact produced in the workshop and subsequently valorized by the institutions and the community.

At an *intermediate-integration level*, the linkage is also mediated by institutional forms of valorization of the participation in the workshop and by functional interchanges between institutions and the workshop (e.g., school credit attributed to some of the workshop activities); the *high-integration level* is characterized by forms of institutional adoptability of the workshop processes and products (e.g., incorporation of some laboratory activities within the activities of local school institutions, municipality, territorial welfare agencies).

Systemic integration serves four purposes. First, it works as an incentive for users. Second, it fosters proximal users' identification with the innovative meanings generated within the workshop setting (see previous, as to the relationship between the identity relevance of practices and the internalization of the meanings underlying them). Third, it operates as an intensifying factor of the criterion of usability of the output, in that it allows the user to experience an increase of their own productive capacity – that is, of the capacity to deliver artifacts that act as resources empowering the capacity of the adult world to (re)signify itself. Finally, and most importantly, systemic integration is the fundamental mechanism through which the conditions of systemic propagation of cultural innovation produced by proximal users are determined. Indeed, it is through the institutional adoption of artifacts that they can operate as a *semiotic virus* capable of spreading the innovative meanings they incorporate (on the concept of the semiotic virus, see Fini & Salvatore, 2018).

A model of community intervention on gambling[2]

This section describes the community intervention strategy to counteract pathological gambling developed as a product of an action research study that one of us recently carried out at the request of the community health agency of a big city in Southern Italy assigned to combat gambling. The request was motivated by the agency's interest in systematizing conceptually and methodologically the community approach to gambling, developed by the team through practices performed over many years.

Theoretical-methodological framework. The action research started from the general idea – underlying the service's community approach – that gambling is not a pathology in itself: it becomes pathological to the extent that it escapes the gambler's capacity for self-regulation (in this regard, see Venuleo et al., 2018). This capacity, on the other hand, is not exclusively individual in nature – on the contrary, it is highly dependent on the social meaning in terms of how gaming (and a gamer) are interpreted within the community. The more gaming is pathologized, that is, interpreted in a polarized way as radical otherness, the less the experience of it can be socialized and become part of community communicative networks, thus elaborated symbolically, explored, and negotiated in both its positive and negative components. As a result of such polarization, gaming ends up being represented in an absolutized key, and, for that reason, it is hard to regulate at the individual level.

Self-regulatory capacities can thus be conceived in a contextual and community key. This means that complementary to the intervention on the individual who has failed in self-regulation (Level of tertiary prevention aimed at pathological gamblers) or at risk of failure (Level of secondary prevention, aimed at at-risk categories), a community intervention (Level of primary prevention) is useful and necessary, aimed at promoting the semiotic resources (semiotic capital) that substantiate less polarized social interpretations of gambling and thus foster individual self-regulation skills.

According to the psycho-semiotic perspective adopted by action research, semiotic capital is produced/processed within and through contexts of social practice operating within the community. The micro-social dynamics that take place within such social practices work as a hub of the meanings through which gambling is interpreted. The promotion of semiotic capital has to be, therefore, carried out as the empowerment of such contexts of social practice and of their capacity to generate innovative meanings concerning gambling and its regulation.

Objective. Based on the previously mentioned theoretical framework, the action research set out to build an intervention model based on the empirical analysis of the sociocultural dynamics of the community, which substantiated players' ability to regulate their own and others' gambling conduct. More specifically, the analysis aimed to:

(a) detect the generalized (worldviews) and specific meanings (e.g., attitudes toward gambling, beliefs about gamblers) involved in the social practices of gambling;
(b) estimate their impact on gambling behavior (forms and intensity) (both at the individual and the community level);
(c) model the mediating/moderating role played by contexts of social practice within which/as a function of which the gambler acts out his/her gambling behavior and its regulation.

It is worth highlighting the essential role that the action research attributed to the last point. Through it, it was intended to go beyond the mere mapping of the semiotic resources that nurture self-regulatory competencies. The identification of the contexts of social practices that mediate the access to and the processing of these resources makes it possible to define a concrete target on which to operate – *where* and *in relation to whom* the promotion of semiotic capital can be pursued.

Preliminary lines of analysis. At the outset, the city territory under the jurisdiction of the agency was made subject to three lines of analysis.

First, the forms and distribution of gaming conduct in the territory were mapped so as to define a system of indicators capable of producing an estimate of the phenomenon in its behavioral, subjective, socioeconomic, and spatial aspects. This line of analysis made it possible to collect relevant information about the *socio-territorial distribution of gambling supply and demand* (e.g., the incidence of different forms and contexts of gaming in the neighborhoods).

Second, a survey was conducted on a representative sample of the city population aimed at detecting representations and attitudes toward gambling, knowledge and perception of the phenomenon, and worldviews (symbolic universes, cf. Chapter 2) active in the cultural milieu. The survey made it possible, among other things, to identify *three representations of gambling* and to estimate their incidence within the population: gambling as an intentional and purpose-oriented activity (*Agency*), gambling as a problematic and ethically sanctionable behavior (*Pathology*), and gambling as a playful activity (*Pleasure*). Another relevant result of this line of analysis was to show that the three representations are influenced by symbolic universes – in particular, the representations of play as Agency and as Pleasure are associated with the symbolic universes expressing a more articulate and future-oriented worldview, while the representation of play as Pathology is preferentially associated with the symbolic universe that has an anomic view of the social context.

Third, the *gaming scenarios* within which individual and social practices of gambling are produced, take shape, and acquire meaning were studied. Since this is the most distinctive line of analysis among those adopted, let us spend a few more words to describe the methodological framework adopted. Scenarios were intended as configurations of socio-organizational characteristics that substantiate a given micro-social format of gaming. Gaming scenarios do not necessarily coincide with gaming places (e.g., Bingo, betting agencies, online gaming): a scenario may characterize transversally a plurality of venues, just as venues of the same type may differ from each other in terms of scenarios. The identification of scenarios was carried out through a grid of analysis developed by the advisors and the agency's team aimed at detecting a plurality of specific psychological, social, material, organizational, and logistical characteristics of gaming places and practices. Examples of the characteristics considered are the presence/absence of a system of filtering/selection of access to the gaming place, characteristics required to access the gaming place, and prevailing relationship structure underlying the gaming practice (monadic, dual, network). The grid of analysis was applied to a sample of gaming practices/places. The data thus collected were processed using a multidimensional analysis procedure (Multiple Correspondence Analysis and Cluster Analysis) designed to identify the ways in which the characteristics detected tend to combine into sufficiently stable configurations. Each configuration thus identified was considered a gaming scenario. Specifically, the main scenarios that emerged from the analysis are the following:

- *impersonal setting*, characterized by individual gaming, regulated by impersonal devices (e.g., bet limit), mediated by those responsible for the place;
- *instrumental container*, characterized by dual (player-to-player) forms of gaming, hosted by logistical and organizational containers that predominantly serve a function of access-filtering;
- *gaming community*, characterized by conditions of access based on players' reputation. In such a scenario, the game is not the end but the mediator of participation in a system of belonging.

The model. The results of the three lines of analysis were related through a structural equation model. More specifically, the model adopted the neighborhood as the unit of analysis and considered the (estimated) incidence of pathological gambling in the neighborhood as the outcome variable. The following characteristics of the neighborhoods (obtained from the second and third lines of preliminary analysis mentioned previously) were used as explanatory variables: a) sociodemographic indicators (education, income, household size); b) incidence of symbolic universes; c) incidence of the three representations of gaming; d) level of social capital; and e) incidence of the three gaming scenarios.

The empirical pattern that emerged from the analysis (see Figure 6.1) showed that gambling is influenced by the social representation of gambling; however, the influence of the social representation of gambling on gambling appears to be not direct but mediated by gaming scenarios. In turn, the social representation is influenced by the more general meanings that substantiate the symbolic universes active within the cultural milieu (the relationship between symbolic universes and gambling representations is both direct and mediated by social capital).

Some of the indicators used in the empirical model are measurements whose accuracy could not be estimated in the context of the action research. The model, therefore, requires further testing. Even with this caution, the model offers empirical support for the contextualist approach to gambling elaborated by the client agency. Moreover, the model represents an empirical validation of the psycho-semiotic form of this approach, focusing on the role of semiotic capital in individual self-regulation of gambling behavior. More importantly, the model highlights the mediating role between semiotic resources and behavior played by the gaming scenarios. This makes the latter a useful methodological and operational anchorage for the design of interventions aimed at promoting competent gaming practices. Indeed, unlike semiotic resources, gaming scenarios have material content – they are located in identifiable places, substantiated by observable social scripts, and endowed

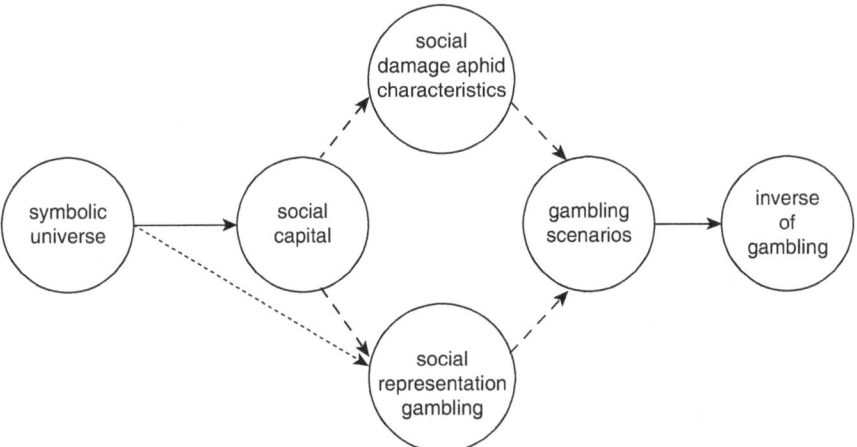

FIGURE 6.1 Model of the psychosocial determinants of gambling

with detectable characteristics. They thus offer themselves as target of actions that can be defined in the modes as well as in the goals pursued in circumstantial and visible ways.

3 Macro-social level

In the two subsections of this section, we present two methodological perspectives – symbolic policy and the promotion of semiotic capital – that can be used to think about psychological interventions at a systemic scale, that is, relating to phenomena that unfold at the macro-social level. At the outset, it is worth highlighting three relevant challenges raised by professional action on this level.

First, by definition, system-scale interventions cannot be conveyed through the mediation of individual/micro-social settings in which the psychologist is directly involved. In other words, in system-scale interventions, the psychologist's body is not the direct driver of the professional action. System-scale interventions do not recognize individuals but populations. System-scale psychological intervention is to psychological action at individual and micro-social scale as the work of the epidemiologist is to that of the physician, as the work of the political economist is to the work of the business manager. The system-scale intervention is thus abstract by definition: lacking the interpersonal substance that is at the heart of psychological theories of technique as well as of the imaginary of psychologists and clients.

Second, and in a complementary way to the previous point, system-scale interventions imply a radicalization of the integrative approach (Carli & Paniccia, 1999) to the professional function. The psychologist engaged in system-scale interventions does not operate directly since, by definition, the regulation/governance of macro-social phenomena is under the responsibility of institutions and agencies. Thus, the function of the psychologist is necessarily that of the prince's advisor: to develop interpretive models and strategies that can enhance the capacity of policies to act on the phenomena/criticalities of interest.

Third, system-scale psychological intervention takes on the typical characteristics of neoprofessionalism (Bosio, 2004; Bosio & Lozza, 2008, 2013, 2018, 2021). Phenomena of the macro-social type cannot be firmly associated with a given professional category. On the contrary, each such phenomenon is an arena where a variety of interpretive and intervention options, each an expression of a professional system, operate in parallel and more or less in conflict with each other. Consequently, on this terrain, psychologists do not have the opportunity to claim/legitimize their role by invoking the psychological nature of the phenomenon on which to intervene. Rather, they find themselves promoting the intervention in a competitive context, where the ability, compared to other professional systems (often endowed with greater media and institutional power; see Chapter 5) to offer functional (effective, viable, plausible) interpretations and solutions counts.

Psychological intervention as a symbolic policy-making function[3]

By symbolic policy, we mean to refer to systematic and purposive actions that an institutional agency (e.g., a public administration) designs and implements with the aim of promoting a change in the way the target population interprets a particular social object. Thus, symbolic policies are a form of public intervention similar to economic, urban, or transportation policies. Like the latter, symbolic policies are aimed at generating resources – in this case, semiotic resources – and regulating their access/distribution within the population. Our thesis is that one of the ways in which psychological intervention can be exercised at the systemic level is to analyze the structure, content, and dynamic of the cultural milieu, aimed at establishing criteria and guidelines for the design, implementation, and verification of symbolic policies. In what follows, we report a case illustrating this mode. This is an action research study that was intended to take on the request of a regional administration in Southern Italy concerning the public valorization of assets confiscated from organized crime.

Objective. The regional administration's interest was in identifying measures to reverse the critical trend of a low civic, social, and economic valorization of assets confiscated from organized crime.

The psychology intervention team took up this request by including it within the conceptual framework of the psycho-semiotic theory. More specifically, it was assumed that the valorization of assets confiscated from organized crime (hereafter, for brevity: confiscated assets) is a function of how individuals and social groups interpret the assets and, more generally, the judicial device of confiscation from crime. This gives rise to the need for institutional agencies engaged with promoting the valorization of confiscated property to equip themselves with a symbolic policy, complementing the regulatory, logistical, managerial, and economic measures that are put in place for this purpose. A symbolic policy is necessary because there can be many ways of interpreting confiscated assets, and those prevailing in the population are not necessarily consistent with the crime-fighting and social promotion objectives that confiscation measures are intended to pursue.

In the context of the valorization of confiscated property, the symbolic policy should be understood as promoting innovative meanings useful in fostering identity and social appropriation of the assets by local communities. In this perspective, as emerged from the joint work with the client system, the function of the symbolic policy of confiscated property aimed at making the confiscated asset a performative symbol of the institutional presence in the territory and of the regenerative capacity of communities – that is to say: a social practice that, in its very exercise, embodies and conveys the sense of the effective and promotional presence of State institutions and the resilience and participation capacity of civil society.

Research. As a first step in fostering the development of a symbolic policy for confiscated property, the advisory team carried out a survey aimed at mapping the social representations of confiscated assets in the regional population. The aim of the survey (carried out on a representative sample of the regional population; N=800) was to provide institutions and stakeholders operating in the region with a knowledge base to be used to design symbolic policy interventions – e.g., involvement of schools, use of social media, communication campaigns; activation of the relational capacities of intermediary bodies; promotion/support of micro-projecting by local administrations and actors; use of the category "confiscated asset" as a brand.

The main findings of the survey can be summarized as follows.

1. Three different social representations of confiscated assets were active in the regional population. A segment of the population consisting of just over one-third of the population (38.38%) represents confiscated assets as an *ideal symbol*, a sign of redemption, justice, the presence of institutions, and legality. This perception is characterized by an affect-laden approach that connotes confiscation as a kind of vexillum: the identity symbol of the reaffirmation of an ethical principle – as such valid, regardless of its actual effectiveness. Another segment, which gathers just under half of the population (49.25%), perceives confiscation as a *potential resource*: a tool that can be useful, whose effectiveness, however, is rendered uncertain by contextual conditions and, in particular, by the incompetence of politicians,

administrators, and those who manage the confiscated assets. Underlying this image are two anchoring meanings: on the one hand, a functional approach, i.e., the idea of confiscation as a tool rather than a sign of identity; on the other, the basically positive assessment of its effectiveness. A third segment, corresponding to about one-fifth of the population (21.38%), sees confiscation as an *ineffective device*: a lever of economic development that nevertheless appears incapable of operating in that sense. This perception shares the same functional view of confiscation as the *potential resource* segment but focused on the economic aspect and expressed a negative assessment of its effectiveness.

2. A relationship between symbolic universes and the social representation of confiscated assets was also found. The three social representations can thus be interpreted as expressions of more general worldviews running through the cultural milieu of the regional society.
3. The three social representations were found to be cross-population rather than characteristics of specific social groups recognizable by reason of factors such as gender, educational level, size of place of residence, and income.
4. The regional population has limited information about the confiscation of property from organized crime: for example, only about 30% of the sample correctly estimates the order of magnitude of the phenomenon.

Implications. The discussion of the results with the various actors of the client system made it possible to develop a set of guidelines for the development of a symbolic policy aimed at the social valorization of confiscated assets. We recall these criteria in what follows, breaking them down into three clusters: A) the characteristics of the sociocultural scenario that is the target of the symbolic policy; B) the symbolic policy objectives that can be pursued by reason of this scenario; and C) possible strategies to be adopted in that perspective.

A) The sociocultural scenario

Interpretive pluralism. Research has shown that within the regional society, confiscated assets are represented according to different meanings, which evidently correspond to different attitudes, judgments, and ways of relating to them. Hence, a need to diversify communication strategies in order to attune them to such pluralism.

Semiotic dependence. The social ways of representing confiscated assets were found not to be autonomous; in other words, these social representations are not construed solely on the basis of information derived (directly or indirectly) from the phenomenon. On the one hand, the research showed that knowledge of the topic is limited and partial within the population. On the other, social representation of confiscated assets depends on superordinate cultural resources, namely on the symbolic universes that are active within the cultural milieu across the social groups that inhabit it. This can constitute an obstacle to a symbolic policy aimed at promoting perceptions of confiscation that are more consistent with the goals of community valorization of confiscated assets since generalized meanings are more widespread and more stable, thus more difficult to change. However, the opposite argument also applies: the development in a progressive sense of social representation of specific social objects is the way institutions can promote the development of semiotic capital – an important strategic goal, especially in socio-territorial contexts characterized by its poor distribution.

Semiotic resources. At an initial level of observation, at least two of the three social representations, corresponding to about 80% of the population, can serve as important semiotic resources. The image of confiscated assets as an *ideal Symbol* is associated with trust and valorization of this device; the image in terms of *potential Resource* qualifies confiscated assets as an effective tool. It is, therefore, to be expected that people who share these two social representations are potentially open to forms of endorsement and/or involvement in processes of community valorization of confiscated assets. It should also be added that even the most critical social representation – *ineffective tool* – associated with about one in five of the population, presents a potential element for development: the negative view it expresses reflects a functional approach to confiscation, understood as a tool at the service of purposes of economic growth. The negative assessment expressed by this social representation is thus not a preconceived closure but the expression of a criterion – economic utility – that can serve as grounds for interaction with those who embrace this social representation.

Criticality. From a complementary point of view, the three social representations all have elements of criticality that limit their ability to foster widespread and entrenched community practices of investment and valorization of confiscated assets. This seems obvious in the case of the *ineffective tool* representation, but it is also true, albeit for different reasons, for the other two social representations. In the case of the *ideal Symbol* representation, confiscation is an expressive act, a symbol: a sign through which to recognize one's own membership of the system of identity or through which to communicate the feeling of impotent rage of those who consider themselves under the yoke of the power of the organized crime, from which they cannot free themselves. As such, the confiscated assets do not belong to the sphere of everyday social life, where elements of reality are part of social practices of utilization and thus are transformed into resources that can be valorized. Transformed into a symbol, the confiscated assets are removed from real life to become an ethical simulacrum to be preserved and celebrated rather than a practice to be performed. In the case of the *potential resource* representation, the critical aspect lies in the protective character that characterizes this image: the confiscated assets are connoted as a form of community resistance against organized crime. Thus interpreted, confiscated assets do not lend themselves to being seen as promotional and participatory or as hubs of community practices. The confiscated assets are conceived as *against*, rather than *for*, something. In other words, it is the exercise of asset *confiscation* as defense and redemption from the threat of organized crime that is foregrounded, while the confiscated *assets* as a lever of development are left in the background.

B) Objective

To integrate functionality and value. In the cultural scenario mapped by the research, the vision of confiscated assets as a value and tool are the opposite extremes of the same dimension of meaning: investment polarized on one aspect *ipso facto* implies the neutralization of the other aspect. However, neither component of meaning appears, by itself, capable of sustaining the community valorization of confiscated assets. On the one hand, the absolutization of the vision of the confiscated assets as a value makes it a simulacrum with which to identify rather than a source of functional utility. On the other hand, the absolutization of the functional value deprives the representation of the confiscated assets of the force of ideality, civicism, and ethical sentiments necessary to motivate the involvement and investment of citizens and thus to fuel community practices of valorization. Thus, the first objective of the symbolic policy should be to bring the poles of this dialectic closer, fusing them – namely, to promote a vision and practice of confiscated assets whose value and identity significance are expressed in their ability to generate functional value (e.g., the success of entrepreneurial and social uses of assets as dynamic symbols of civic resistance to organized crime) and, at the same time, whose functional significance is exercised through their symbolic value (e.g., brand value of productive activities associated with confiscated assets).

C) Strategies

Enhancing the autonomy of perceptions. A general strategy suggested by the analysis is to foster the progressive autonomy of perceptions from superordinate beliefs (see previous). The more people interpret confiscated assets because of the aspects concerning them, the more innovations introduced in this area will be able to foster changes in ways of perceiving and, therefore, acting. Enhancing autonomy requires systematic actions to inform and promote the visibility of the confiscated assets system so that this social object can progressively acquire representational centrality within the collective imagination. It also requires the adoption of forms of communication capable of activating not only the cognitive dimension but also the affective component of citizenship; this is because it is only under this condition that innovative meanings can remain active in the collective representational field without being assimilated/neutralized by hegemonic superordinate meanings.

Investing in performative vectors. Complementary to what has been proposed previously, innovative meanings must be conveyed primarily in performative terms (see Chapters 2 and 3). In other words, innovation in ways of signifying confiscated assets does not so much come through explicit discourses and norms as through the spread and consolidation of emblematic social practices that convey in their very configuration the meanings they intend to promote. The declarative, explicit communication of meanings follows as a reflective practice on what has already been performatively exercised and thereby activated. From this point of view, the design, activation, validation, and dissemination of prototypes of social practices that reverse patterns of utilization of confiscated assets, capable of nurturing community valorization, is extremely useful.

Strengthening the rooting of assets in the community fabric. The territorial community is probably the central resource in the process of valorization of confiscated assets. There is extensive literature in support of the thesis that the integration of functionality and value comes about through the mediation of community relations. However, the enrooting of assets in the community fabric requires that a dynamic balance be established between appropriation of the asset by the lifeworlds – that is, by groups of people who share and give existential meaning and identity value to their investment in assets – and institutional regulation of this process. Without an appropriation, the good would not be laden with subjective and identity value, ending up operating, at the limit, as a mere logistical container of economic and functional activities devoid of identity value. On the other hand, in the absence of the regulatory function exercised by institutions, lifeworlds, given their intrinsic self-referentiality and centering on the present, are unable to guarantee the systematic investment required for the valorization of assets in the medium term. The fundamental challenge is to identify organizational and public intervention models that can generate intermediate processes, that is, processes within which lifeworlds and institutions can interact and transform the inherent tension between meaning and functionality into a generative dialectic (see the next subsection, Section 3.2).

Promotion of semiotic capital and intermediate processes

In a number of recent papers (Cordella et al., 2023; Cremaschi et al., 2021; Salvatore et al., 2018, 2019b, 2021; Salvatore, De Luca Picione et al., 2022), the psycho-semiotic model underlying this book has been used to construct an interpretive key to the socio-institutional crisis that runs through the contemporary world (more specifically, Western European societies). At the heart of this interpretation is the thesis that the many macro-social criticalities we face – from the disarticulation between lifeworlds and institutions (e.g., the educational conflict between family and school system) to the crisis of functionality and trust in welfare systems, from gender violence to Euroscepticism, from political and ideological polarization to xenophobia, from the proliferation of fake news to the weakening of democratic institutions, from fatalism toward climate change to the re-emergence of the specter of nuclear conflict – however different in their content and consequences, are *manifestations of a global sociocultural dynamic of generalized impoverishment of the semiotic capital*. This dynamic is fueled by the profound social and institutional transformations induced by globalization and further exacerbated by the crisis, first economic and then socio-institutional, that has infested advanced capitalist Western societies in the last decades.

The impoverishment of the cultural milieus of European societies has resulted in an overall weakening of the civic and institutional infrastructure that has long operated as a constant framework of meaning at the foundation of the relations among individuals and among peoples. What is taking place is an *anthropological drift* – a radical change in the ways of feeling, thinking, and acting, which make obsolete institutional frameworks, interpretive categories, and modes of relations among individuals and among social groups – in a word: what has nurtured the forms of life that until the recent past acted as the scaffolding of subjectivity and sociality is dissolving (Mazzoni, 2015).

How do we counter such a drift? Can psychology offer a contribution in this regard?

Framed on an extensive analysis of the sociocultural dynamics of European societies (Salvatore et al., 2019a, 2019b) and on the guidelines elaborated on the basis of such an analysis (Re.Cri.Re. Consortium, 2018), the works mentioned previously have tried to answer these questions. They proposed theoretical and empirical arguments in support of the need to combine two systemic strategies.

On the one hand, action is needed to counter the current drift. This inevitably passes through structural interventions to reduce the systemic uncertainty that characterizes the globalized world. Indeed, uncertainty can be seen as the fundamental source of semiotic impoverishment, as it fuels socio-cognitive responses characterized by simplified, affect-laden forms of feeling, thinking, and acting (Salvatore et al., 2021, 2023). Reducing uncertainty requires working as much on the social and economic factors that fuel it – for example, the progressive growth of inequality (Piketty, 2013/2014), the opacity of institutional and socioeconomic regulatory mechanisms, the deterritorialization of decision-making processes – as on enhancing the capacities of individuals and collective actors to construct interpretive frames capable of operating as buffers against the instability, unpredictability and limited representability of social dynamics (Salvatore et al., 2019a).

On the other – and here, the contribution of the psychological function may prove to be central – work needs to be done to create the socio-institutional conditions useful for fostering a new phase of semiotic capital accumulation. A central role, in this perspective, is played by *intermediate processes*. Intermediate processes are social practices conveyed by meaningful interpersonal ties. Thus, intermediate processes retain the characteristics typical of lifeworlds – namely, the sphere of everyday intersubjective practices that bind the individual to close others (family members, friends, neighbors), whose meaning is assumed unreflectively, given in the immediacy of experience. At the same time, however, intermediate processes are oriented toward the pursuit of meta-interpersonal purposes – objectives of a systemic nature or public value. These purposes operate as a superordinate criterion that limits the inherent self-referentiality of lifeworlds. The intermediate process, then, solicits the expression of interpersonal subjectivity – the affective and simplified modes of feeling, thinking, and acting associated with it – and, at the same time, expresses toward such subjectivity a demand for regulation, constraint, and finalization. In other words, in an intermediate process, actors cannot simply wait for Godot – they are called upon to perform a third function, namely a function that works as a superordinate point of view that makes possible the regulation and finalization of lifeworlds.

All of this leads to the conclusion that in an intermediate process, the meanings that preside over the representation of the systemic and public dimension of socio-institutional scenarios – in other words, the semiotic resources that make norms, commons, the sense of living as a collective fact thinkable – meet with the lifeworlds, thus "filling" themselves with subjectivity and unreflective immediacy. It is this possibility that makes intermediate processes *hubs of semiotic capital* – i.e., settings of social practice within which innovative interpretations of the interpersonal, social, and institutional worlds can be generated and, at the same time, made able to foster in people the experience of the public dimension as a salient, meaningful and vital object, existentially dense – as such an emotional, cognitive, and behavioral regulator.

In Western societies, at least until the last two decades of the last century, the transitional dynamic between subjectivity and the public sphere occurred through social entities (unions, parties, associations) that served as containers of intermediate processes. These entities fulfilled a key role in mediating between lifeworlds and institutions, constituting themselves as the neuralgic scaffolding of the democracies that emerged in the aftermath of World War II (Ardigò, 1982). In the last 30 years, we have witnessed the progressive weakening of such intermediate bodies, a dynamic that can be interpreted both as the main distal cause of the impoverishment of semiotic capital and as a consequence of the sociopolitical crisis associated with that impoverishment (Russo et al., 2020). Think, in this sense, of the substantial disappearance, in many Western democracies, of political parties as collective subjects capable of generating a sense of identity for large sectors of society. Again, consider the personalization of political discourse around charismatic leaders and the increasingly widespread disaffection with the institutional mechanisms and practices of concertation and synthesis of the complex network of pluralist interests in areas ranging from labor relations to the functioning of public administrations. Consider the growing tendency of families to absolutize their educational demand with respect to school institutions, indicative of the inability to recognize the thirdness of this institution, its function of serving a superordinate public function with respect to the demand for reproduction inherent in the lifeworlds.

In the context of contemporary societies, it is, therefore, difficult to believe that the production of semiotic capital can be pursued in the form in which it was realized in a phase of history now behind us. This is the reason why we consider it appropriate to refer to *processes* rather than intermediary *bodies*. Imagining intervention strategies based on the idea of rebuilding parties, unions, and the fabric of religious and civic associationism that characterized society several decades ago is just as realistic as thinking of coping with climate change by replacing cars and airplanes with horses. Intermediation should be understood in dynamic rather than structural terms. Intermediary processes are contingent networks of social practices, triggered and nurtured by policies of different scales (from the territorial to the transnational level), operating within or across domains of activity (education, health, transportation, inclusion), endowed with variable time horizons (very short, short, medium term), designed to operate by means of participatory settings where lifeworlds and systemic instances can meet with each other, opening up to the possibility of mutual dialecticization.

An example of designing an intermediate process is provided by a proposal that one of us recently helped to design. In previous years, the municipal administration of a city in Northeast Italy had invested many resources in the implementation of a program of interventions aimed at reducing the risk of flooding, to which that territorial area is particularly exposed. The program consisted of the implementation of a widespread network of small devices set up within the areas owned by members of the community (e.g., vegetable gardens, plots intended for cultivation), as a whole, designed to enhance the soil's capacity to absorb water (e.g., secondary runoff channels). The land preservation policy was thus characterized by the direct involvement of the local community, which responded positively, providing active and proactive cooperation in the implementation of the interventions to contribute decisively to the positive infrastructural results of the program.

The proposal addressed to the administration described in what follows starts from the framework outlined previously. More specifically, the recognition of how community participation in land preservation policy had been limited to the engineering dimension relates to the construction and maintenance of devices. This approach, not at all unusual, reflects a general logic of public intervention that leads only the functional and structural aspects of policies to be seen while in the background, the semiotic resources are involved in interventions (Andriola et al., 2019; Cremaschi et al., 2021). In short, public policies are generally conceived as *interventions on objects* rather than *with subjects*.

Based on the considerations summarized previously, the psychological advisor identified a potential for further development in the land policy implemented by the municipal administration, seeing in it the opportunity to operate as a vector of an intermediate process involving broad segments of the local community. Concretely, this can be done by involving the local community in the permanent action of risk monitoring and management through the definition of an institutionalized participatory device (e.g., a permanent civic committee to be activated at the municipality), which would be entrusted with the function of making proposals to the municipal administration, regarding land control and prevention measures – e.g., observation and intervention system on water flows, procedures and ways of controlling the efficiency of runoff devices, and the definition and updating of plans for the protection of the population and facilities.

In terms of the discussion proposed in this subsection, what we are envisaging is the activation of an intermediate process: a local and contingent setting – i.e., activated as a result of a specific initiative with a circumscribed scope of competencies – in which actors participate from within and because of their own private sphere – i.e., motivated by their own interest, concerns for themselves, their families and their property. At the same time, such a space is constituted as an arena that calls on participants to adopt a systemic, superordinate point of view, broader than the particular one: the point of view defined by the institutionalized participatory device's role of serving the interests of the city as a whole.

Notes

1 This section is a reworking of the paper: Andreassi, S., & Salvatore S. (2021). *Notes on the 1, 2, 3 Star Association intervention model* [Unpublished manuscript]. Department of Dynamic, Clinical and Health Psychology, Sapienza University of Rome. We express our gratitude to our colleague Silvia Andreassi, aware of how much the ideas elaborated in the manuscript reflect her contributions. We are grateful to the 1, 2, 3 Star Association of Rome, the client of the consultancy of which the paper is one of the results, for allowing us to use the material.

2 This section reports on action research commissioned by the Dipartimento Dipendenze, Azienda Sanitaria Locale NA/1, Naples (Italy). The action research was carried out in collaboration with colleagues of the agency. The results and ideas presented here owe much to their contributions and the mixture of expertise and passion that characterizes them.

3 This section is a reworking of the paper: Salvatore S., & Cozzolino, M. (2020). *Perceptions of the confiscation of property from organized crime in Campania: Analysis and criteria for the definition of community enhancement policies for confiscated property* [Unpublished manuscript]. Department of Human, Philosophical and Educational Sciences, University of Salerno and European Institute of Cultural Analysis for Policies.

REFERENCES

Albanesi, C., Rochira, A., & Barbieri, I. (2021). Il senso di comunità. In C. Arcidiacono, N. De Piccoli, T. Mannarini, & E. Marta (Eds.), *Psicologia di comunità: Prospettive e concetti chiave* [Community psychology: Perspective and key concepts]. Franco Angeli.

Andreassi, S., Signore, F., Cordella, B., De Dominicis, S., Gennaro, A., Iuso, S., Kerušauskaitė, S., Kosic, A., Mannarini, T., Reho, M., Rocchi, G., Rochira, A., Scharfbillig, M., & Salvatore, S. (2023). Identity and symbolic universes in voting behavior: A study of the Italian society. *Psychology Hub, 2,* 69–80. https://doi.org/10.13133/2724-2943/17900

Andriola, V., Been, W., Cremaschi, M., Fini, V., Matsopoulos, A., Willet, J., & Salvatore, S. (2019). Policies and sensemaking. In S. Salvatore, V. Fini, T. Mannarini, J. Valsiner, & G. A. Veltri (Eds.), *Symbolic universes in time of (post)crisis: The future of European societies* (pp. 271–291). Springer.

Angus, L. E., & McLeod, J. (Eds.). (2004). *The handbook of narrative and psychotherapy: Practice, theory and research.* Sage Publishing.

Antonucci, L. A., Bellantuono, L., Kleinbub, J. R., Lella, A., Palmieri, A., & Salvatore, S. (2022). The harmonium model and its unified system view of psychopathology: A validation study by means of a convolutional neural network. *Scientific Reports, 12,* 21789. https://doi.org/10.1038/s41598-022-26054-9

Appadurai, A. (2013). *The future as cultural fact: Essays on the global condition.* Verso Book.

Ardigò, A. (1982). *Crisi di governabilità e mondi vitali* [Crisis of governance and lifeworlds]. Nuova Universale Cappelli.

Associazione Italiana di Psicologia. (2019). *I problemi della "sicurezza": L'impatto psicologico e psicosociale della legge 132/2018* [*Problem of "security": The psychological and psychosocial impact of the low 132/2018*]. www.aipass.org/aip-immigrazione-e-sicurezza

Baerveldt, C., & Verheggen, T. (2012). Enactivism. In J. Valsiner (Ed.), *Oxford handbook of culture and psychology* (pp. 165–190). Oxford University Press.

Banfield, E. C. (1958). *The moral basis of a backward society*. The Free Press.

Barrett, L. F. (2006). Solving the emotion paradox: Categorization and the experience of emotion. *Personality and Social Psychology Review, 10,* 20–46.

Barrett, L. F., & Lindquist, K. A. (2008). The embodiment of emotion. In G. R. Semin & E. R. Smith (Eds.), *Embodied grounding: Social, cognitive, affective, and neuroscientific approaches* (pp. 237–262). Cambridge University Press.

Barrett, L. F., & Russell, J. A. (1999). The structure of current affect: Controversies and emerging consensus. *Current Directions in Psychological Science, 8,* 10–14.

Barsalou, L. W. (1999). Perceptual symbol systems. *Behavioral and Brain Sciences, 22,* 577–660.

Barsalou, L. W. (2008). Grounded cognition. *Annual Review of Psychology, 59,* 617–645.

Barsalou, L. W. (2011). Integrating Bayesian analysis and mechanistic theories in grounded cognition. *Behavioral and Brain Sciences, 34,* 191–192.

Bateson, G. (1972). *Steps to an ecology of mind: Collected essays in anthropology, psychiatry, evolution, and epistemology*. University of Chicago Press.

Bellini, L., & Maestripieri, L. (2018). Professions within, between and beyond: Varieties of professionalism in a globalising world. *Cambio, 8*(16), 5–14.

Benedict, R. (1935). *Patterns of culture*. Routledge & Kegan Pvt. Ltd.

Berger, P., & Luckman, T. (1966). *The social construction of reality: A treatise in the sociology of knowledge*. Open Road.

Berry, J. W., Poortinga, Y. H., Segall, M. H., & Dasen, P. R. (2002). *Cross-cultural psychology: Research and applications* (2nd ed.). Cambridge University Press.

Bickhard, M. H. (2009). Interactivism: A manifesto. *New Ideas in Psychology, 27,* 85–89.

Boas, F. (1911). *The mind of the primitive man*. The Macmillan Company.

Bonazzi, G. (1989). *Storia del pensiero organizzativo* [History of the organizational thought]. Franco Angeli.

Bordin, E. S. (1979). The generalizability of the psychoanalytic concept of the working alliance. *Psychotherapy: Theory, Research & Practice, 16*(3), 252–260.

Borghi, A. M., Binkofski, F., Castelfranchi, C., Cimatti, F., Scorolli, C., & Tummolini, L. (2017). The challenge of abstract concepts. *Psychological Bulletin, 143*(3), 263–292.

Bosio, A. C. (2004). Introduzione: Verso un marketing delle professioni? [Introduction: Towards a marketing of professions?]. *Micro & Macro Marketing, 1,* 103–116.

Bosio, A. C., & Lozza, E. (2008). Lo stato e il futuro delle professioni psicologiche nella prospettiva degli psicologi del Lazio [Current state and the future of the psychological professions in accordance with the standpoint of psychologists from Lazio]. In G. Ponzio (Ed.), *La psicologia e il mercato del lavoro: Una nuova professione destinata al precariato? Le ricerche dell'osservatorio Mercato del Lavoro* (pp. 83–107). Franco Angeli.

Bosio, A. C., & Lozza, E. (2013). Professionalizzazione della psicologia e professioni psicologiche: Il percorso e le prospettive in Italia [Professionalization of psychology and psychological professions: Trajectory and perspective in Italy]. *Giornale Italiano di Psicologia, 40*(4), 675–690.

Bosio, A. C., & Lozza, E. (2018). Professionalizzare: Missione (im-)possibile per l'università? [Professionalize: (Im)possible mission for the university?]. *Vita e Pensiero, 6,* 117–126.

Bosio, A. C., & Lozza, E. (2021). La costruzione sociale delle professioni psicologiche in Italia: Percorsi e agenda building [The social construction of the psychological professions: Pathways and agenda bulding]. *Giornale Italiano di Psicologia, 48*(2), 367–386.

Bourdieu, P. (1977). *Outline of a theory of practice* (Vol. 16). Cambridge University Press. (Original work published in French, Droz 1973)

Bowlby, J. (1969). *Attachment and loss: Vol. I. Attachment*. Hogarth.

Bruner, J. (1990). *Acts of meaning*. Harvard University Press.

Bucci, W. (1997). *Psychoanalysis and cognitive science*. The Guildford Press.

Bühler, K. (1990). *Theory of language: The representational function of language*. John Benjamins Publishing Co. (Original work published 1934)

Butera, F. (1991). *Il castello e la rete* [The castle and the network]. Franco Angeli.

Carli, R. (1987a). L'analisi della domanda [The analysis of the demand]. *Rivista di Psicologia Clinica, 1*(1), 38–53.

Carli, R. (1987b). *Psicologia clinica* [Clinical psychology]. UTET.

Carli, R. (1988). Per una teoria della tecnica [For a theory of technique]. *Rivista di Psicologia Clinica, 2*, 6–21.

Carli, R. (a cura di). (1993). *L'analisi della domanda in psicologia clinica* [The analysis of the demand in clinical psychology]. Giuffrè.

Carli, R. (1997). L'analisi della domanda rivisitata [The analysis of the demand revised]. *Psicologia Clinica, 2*(1), 5–21.

Carli, R. (2007). Notes on the report. *Rivista di Psicologia Clinica, 2*, 181–200.

Carli, R., & Paniccia, R. M. (1981). *Psicosociologia delle organizzazioni e delle istituzioni* [Psychosociology of organizations and institutions]. Il Mulino.

Carli, R., & Paniccia, R. M. (1999). *Psicologia della formazione* [Psychology of training]. Il Mulino.

Carli, R., & Paniccia, R. M. (2003). *Analisi della domanda – Teoria e intervento in psicologia clinica* [The analysis of the demand: Theory and intervention in clinical psychology]. Il Mulino.

Carrettero, M., & Kriger, M. (2011). Historical representations and conflicts about indigenous people as national identities. *Culture & Psychology, 17*(2), 177–195.

Carr-Saunders, A. M. (1928). *Professions: Their organization and place in society* [Herbert Spencer lecture]. Clarendon Press.

Caspi, A., Houts, R. M., Belsky, D. W., Goldman-Mellor, S. J., Harrington, H., Israel, S., & Moffitt, T. E. (2014). The p factor: One general psychopathology factor in the structure of psychiatric disorders? *Clinical Psychological Science, 2*(2), 119–137.

Ciavolino, E., Salvatore, S., Mossi, P., & Vernai, M. (2017). Quality and prosumership. Proserv: A new tool for measuring the customer satisfaction. *International Journal of Business and Society, 18*(3), 409–426.

Cionini, L. (2001). *Psicoterapie: Modelli a confronto* [Psychotherapies: Models in comparisons]. Carocci.

Circolo del Cedro. (1992). La competenza psicologico-clinica: Riflessioni e proposte del Circolo del Cedro [The competence for clinical psychology: Notes and proposals by Circolo del Cedro]. *Rivista di Psicologia Clinica, 6*, 6–37.

Clark, A. (2005). Beyond the flesh: Some lessons from a mole cricket. *Artificial Life, 11*(1–2), 233–244.

Cole, M. (1996). *Cultural psychology: A once and future discipline*. Harvard University Press.

Coleman, J. S. (1988). Social capital in the creation of human capital. *American Journal of Sociology*, *94*(Suppl), S95–S120.

Corballis, M. C. (2011). *The recursive mind: The origins of human language, thought, and civilization*. Princeton University Press.

Cordella, B., Grasso, M., & Pennella, A. R. (2004). *Metodologia dell'intervento in psicologia clinica* [Methodology of intervention in clinical psychology]. Carocci.

Cordella, B., Grasso, M., & Pennella, A. R. (2022). *Metodologia dell'intervento in Psicologia clinica: Nuova edizione* [Methodology of intervention in clinical psychology: New edition]. Carocci.

Cordella, B., & Salvatore, S. (2021). Il valore della psicologia [The value of psychology]. *Giornale Italiano di Psicologia*, *48*, 383–388.

Cordella, B., Signore, F., Andreassi, S., De Dominicis, S., Gennaro, A., Iuso, S., Mannarini, T., Kerusauskaite, S., Kosic, A., Reho, M., Rochira, A., Rocchi, G., & Salvatore, S. (2023). How socio-institutional contexts and cultural worldviews relate to COVID-19 acceptance rates: A representative study in Italy. *Social Science & Medicine*, *320*, 115671. https://doi.org/10.1016/j.socscimed.2023.115671

Cornoldi, C. (1995). *Metacognizione e apprendimento* [Metacognition and learning]. Il Mulino.

Cremaschi, M., Fioretti, C., Mannarini, M., & Salvatore, S. (2021). *Culture and policy-making: Pluralism, performativity and semiotic capital*. Springer.

Crozier, M., & Friedberg, E. (1977). *L'actour et le systeme: Les contraintes de l'action colective* [The actor and the system: The constraints of the collective action]. Edition de Seuil.

Cuccio, V., & Gallese, V. (2018). A Peircean account of concepts: Grounding abstraction in phylogeny through a comparative neuroscientific perspective. *Philosophical Transaction of the Royal Society: Biological Sciences*, *373*.

de la Sablonnière, R. (2017). Toward a psychology of social change: A typology of social change. *Frontiers in Psychology*, *8*, 397.

De Luca Picione, R. (2021). Models of semiotic borders in psychology and their implications: From rigidity of separation to topological dynamics of connectivity. *Theory & Psychology*, *31*(5), 729–745.

De Luca Picione, R., & Salvatore, S. (2023). Mind is movement: We need more than static representations to understand it. In J. Valsiner (Ed.), *Farewell variables* (pp. 137–157). Information Age Publishing.

De Rosa, A. (Ed.). (2013). *Social respresentation in "social arena"*. Routledge.

de Saussure, F. (1977). *Course in general linguistics* (W. Baskin, Trans.). Fontana/Collins. (Original work published 1916)

Di Maria, F. (2005). *Psicologia per la politica: Metodi e pratiche* [Psychology for polity: Methods and practice]. Franco Angeli.

Di Maria, F. (2021). Per una psicologia psicologica [For a psychological psychology]. *Rivista di Psicologia Clinica*, *16*(2), 24–29.

Doise, W., Mugny, G., & Pérez, J. A. (1998). The social construction of knowledge: Social marking and socio-cognitive conflict (G. Duveen, Trans.). In U. Flick (Ed.), *The psychology of the social* (pp. 77–90). Cambridge University Press.

Douglas, M. (1986). *How institutions think*. Syracuse University Press.

Douglas, M., & Wildavsky, A. B. (1982). *Risk and culture: An essay on the selection of technical and environmental dangers*. University of California Press.

Eco, U. (1975). *A theory of semiotic*. Indiana University Press.

Elchardus, M., & Spruyt, B. (2016). Populism, persistent republicanism and declinism: An empirical analysis of populism as a thin ideology. *Government and Opposition*, *51*(1), 111–133.

Engel, A. K., Friston, K. J., & Kragic, D. (2015). Introduction: Where's the action? In A. K. Engel, K. J. Friston, & D. Kragic (Eds.), *The pragmatic turn: Toward action-oriented views in cognitive science* (pp. 1–15). MIT Press.

Etchegoyen, R. H. (2005). *Foundational of psychoanalytic technique*. Routledge.

Evans, V., & Green, M. (2006). *Cognitive linguistics. An introduction*. Edinburgh University Press.

Evetts, J. (2003). The sociological analysis of professionalism: Occupational change in the modern world. *International Sociology*, *18*(2), 395–415.

Ferro, A. (2005). Which reality in the psychoanalytic session? *Psychoanalytic Quarterly*, *74*, 421–442.

Fini, V., & Salvatore, S. (2018). The fuel and the engine: A general semio-cultural psychological framework for social intervention. In S. Schliewe, N. Chaudhary, & P. Marsico (Eds.), *Cultural psychology of intervention in the globalized world* (pp. 23–47). Information Age Publishing.

Foa, R. S., & Mounk, Y. (2016). The democratic disconnect. *Journal of Democracy*, *27*(3), 5–17. https://doi.org/10.1353/jod.2016.0049

Fodor, J. A. (1983). *The modularity of mind: An essay on faculty psychology*. The MIT Press.

Fornari, F. (1979). *I fondamenti di una teoria psicoanalitica del linguaggio* [Foundation of a psychoanalytic theory of language]. Boringhieri.

Fornari, F. (1983). *La lezione freudiana* [The Freudian lessons]. Feltrinelli.

Freda, M. F., Esposito, G., & Famiglietti, M. F. (2013). La competenza a resocontare nella formazione alla psicologia clinica: Un'indagine qualitativa [The competence to report in the training to clinical psychology: A qualitative study]. *Psicologia Scolastica*, *11*(1), 47–65.

Freda, M. F., & Oberti, A. (2007). Support as a source of meanings: Report of an intervention with a parents' association. *Rivista di Psicologia Clinica*, *3*, 339–353.

Freud, S. (1953). The interpretation of dreams. In J. Strachey (Ed. & Trans.), *The standard edition of the complete psychological works of Sigmund Freud* (Vol. 4–5). The Hogarth Press and the Institute of Psycho-analysis. (Original work published 1900)

Friston, K. (2010). The free-energy principle: A unified brain theory? *Nature Reviews Neuroscience*, *11*(2), 127.

Fronterotta, F., Di Letizia, R., & Salvatore, S. (2018). Processual monism: A fresh look at the mind-body problem. *Minds and Matter*, *16*(2), 167–194.

Gagliardi, P. (a cura di). (1986). *Le imprese come culture: Nuove prospettive di analisi organizzativa* [Companies as cultures: New perspective of organizational analysis]. ISEDI.

Gaj, N. (2009). Verso un modello unificato in psicologia clinica. Un'analisi storico epistemologica sullo sviluppo della disciplina [Towards a unified model in clinical psychology: An historical-epistemological analysis on the development of the discipline]. *Ricerche di Psicologia*, 1–22.

Gallagher, S. (2005). *How the body shapes the mind*. Oxford University Press.

Gamson, W. A. (1988). Political discourse and collective action. In B. Klandermans (Ed.), *From structure to action: Comparing social movement research across cultures* (pp. 219–244). JAI Press.

Geertz, C. (1983). *Local knowledge: Further essays in interpretative anthropology*. Basic Books.

Gennaro, A., Goncalves, M., Mendes, I., Ribeiro, A., & Salvatore, S. (2011). Dynamics of sense-making and development of the narrative in the clinical exchange. *Research in Psychotherapy: Psychopathology Process and Outcome, 14*(1), 90–120 [online journal]. www.researchinpsychotherapy.net

Gergen, K. J. (1985). The social constructionist movement in modern psychology. *American Psychologist, 40*(3), 266–275.

Gergen, K. J. (1999). *An invitation to social construction*. Sage Publishing.

Giannone, F., & Lo Verso, G. (1998). I presupposti epistemologici [Epistemological assumptions]. In S. Di Nuovo, G. Lo Verso, M. Di Blasi, & F. Giannone (a cura di), *Valutare le psicoterapie: La ricerca italiana* (pp. 17–39). Franco Angeli.

Gillespie, A. (2010). The intersubjective nature of symbols. In B. Wagoner (Ed.), *Symbolic transformation: The mind in movement through culture and society* (pp. 23–37). Routledge.

Graffigna, G. (2021). *Esitanti: Quello che la pandemia ci ha insegnato sulla psicologia della prevenzione* [Hesitating: What the pandemic taught about the psychology of prevention]. Il Pensiero Scientifico Editore.

Grassi, R. (2004). Costruendo narrazioni [Constructing narration]. In G. Montesarchio, R. Grassi, E. Marzella, & C. Venuleo (Eds.), *Indizi di colloquio* (pp. 65–93). Franco Angeli.

Grasso, M., Cordella, B., & Pennella, A. R. (2003). *L'intervento in psicologia clinica* [The intervention in clinical psychology]. Carocci.

Grasso, M., Cordella, B., & Pennella, A. R. (2016). *L'intervento in psicologia clinica: Nuova edizione* [The intervention in clinical psychology: New edition]. Carocci.

Grasso, M., & Salvatore, S. (1997). *Pensiero e decisionalità: Contributo alla critica della prospettiva individualista in psicologia* [Tought and decision-making: Contribution to the critique of the individualist perspective in psychology]. Franco Angeli.

Grasso, M., & Stampa, P. (2011). Psychological normality, psychopathology and evidence-based psychotherapy: Are we so sure "we're not in Kansas anymore"? In S. Salvatore & T. Zittoun (Eds.), *Cultural psychology and psychoanalysis: Pathways to synthesis* (pp. 225–278). Information Age Publishing.

Grasso, M., & Stampa, P. (2014). *L'inconscio non abita più qui: Psicologia clinica e psicoterapia nella società dell'illusione di massa* [The unconscious does not live here anymore: Clinical psychology and psychotherapy in the society of the mass illusion]. Franco Angeli.

Grazzani, I., & Brockmeier, J. (2019). Language games and social cognition: Revisiting Bruner. *Integrative Psychological and Behavioral Science, 53*, 602–610.

Green, C. D. (2015). Why psychology isn't unified, and probably never will be. *Review of General Psychology, 19*(3), 207–214.

Greenberg, J., & Arndt, J. (2012). Terror management theory. In P. A. M. Van Lange, A. W. Kruglanski, & E. Tory Higgins (Eds.), *Handbook of theories of social psychology* (pp. 398–415). Sage Publishing.

Greenwood, E. (1957). Attributes of a profession. *Social Work, 2*(3), 45–55.

Guidi, M., Fini, V., & Salvatore, S. (2015a). The school system: A survey on the school principals' models of signification. *Rivista di Psicologia Clinica, 10*(1), 131–166. www.rivistadipsicologiaclinica.it

Guidi, M., Venuleo, C., & Salvatore, S. (2015b). The meaning of being at school: The models of signification of the school context in a sample of high school students. *Rivista di Psicologia Clinica, 10*(1), 57–93. www.rivistadipsicologiaclinica.it

Harmon, D. J. (2020). Arguments and institutions. In P. Haack, J. Sieweke, & L. Wessel (Eds.), *Microfoundations of institutions* (Vol. 65B, pp. 3–22). Emerald.

Harré, R., & Gillett, G. (1994). *The discursive mind.* Sage Publishing.

Harré, R., & Sammut, G. (2013). What lies between? In G. Sammut, P. Daanen, & F. M. Moghaddam (Eds.), *Understanding the self and others: Explorations in intersubjectivity and interobjectivity* (pp. 15–30). Routledge.

Harrison, L. E., & Huntington, S. P. (Eds.). (2000). *Culture matters: How values shape human progress.* Basic Books.

Heft, H. (2013). Environment, cognition, and culture: Reconsidering the cognitive map. *Journal of Environmental Psychology, 33,* 14–25.

Heine, S. J. (2016). *Cultural psychology* (3rd ed.). Norton.

Henriques, G. (2011). *A new unified theory of psychology.* Springer.

Hermans, H. J. M., & Hermans-Jansen, E. (1995). *Self-narratives: The construction of meaning in psychotherapy.* The Guilford.

Hirose, I., & Olson, J. (Eds.). (2015). *The Oxford handbook of value theory.* Oxford University Press.

Hochschild, R. A. (2016). *Strangers in their own land: Anger and mourning on the American right. A journey to the heart of our political divide.* The New Press.

Hoffman, I. Z. (1998). *Ritual and spontaneity in the psychoanalytic process.* The Analytic Press Inc.

Huntington, S. S. (2000). Forewords: Culture counts. In L. Harrison & S. P. Huntington (Eds.), *Culture matters* (pp. xiii–xvi). Basic Books.

Iannaccone, A. (2010). *Le condizioni sociali del pensiero* [The social condition of the thought]. Unicopli.

Iannaccone, A., & Ghodbane, I. (2005). La "ricerca del significato" nel contesto universitario; il mestiere di studente [The search for meaning in the university context; the job of student]. In T. Mannarini, A. Perucca, & S. Salvatore (a cura di), *Quale psicologia per la scuola del futuro?* (pp. 37–57). Edizioni Carlo.

Inglehart, R. (1971). The silent revolution in Europe. Intergenerational change in post-industrial societies. *The American Political Science Review, 65*(4), 991–1017.

Inglehart, R., & Norris, P. (2017). Trump and the populist authoritarian parties: The silent revolution in reverse. *Perspectives on Politics, 15*(2), 443–454.

Inglehart, R., & Welzel, C. (2005). *Modernization, cultural change, and democracy: The human development sequence.* Cambridge University Press. https://doi.org/10.1017/CBO9780511790881 PMID:11120488

Ivaldi, A. (2016). *Il trattamento dei disturbi dissociativi e di personalità: Teoria e clinica del modello relazionale fondato sui sistemi motivazionali* [The treatment of the dissociative and personality diseases: Theory and clinic of the relational model based on the motivational systems]. Franco Angeli.

Jason, L. A. (2013). *Principles of social change.* Oxford University Press.

Johnson-Laird, P. N. (1983). *Mental models: Towards a cognitive science of language, inference, and consciousness.* Harvard University Press.

Kahneman, D. (2003). A perspective on judgment and choice: Mapping bounded rationality. *American Psychologist, 58,* 697–720.

Kazdin, A. (2008). Unity: Psychology's immunity booster. *Monitor on Psychology.* www.apa.org/monitor/2008/03/pc

Kimble, G. A. (1990). Mother nature's bag of tricks is small. *Psychological Science, 1,* 36–41.

Kirshner, L. A. (2010). Between Winnicott and Lacan: Reclaiming the subject of psychoanalysis. *American Imago, 67,* 331–351.

Klein, M. (1967). *Contribution to psychoanalysis, 1921–1945.* McGraw-Hill.

Klein, N. (1999). *No logo, taking aim at the brand bullies.* Picador.

Kleinbub, J., Testolin, A., Palmieri, A., & Salvatore, S. (2021). The phase space of meaning model of psychopathology: A computer simulation modeling study. *PLOS One, 16*(4), e0249320.

Koltko-Rivera, M. E. (2004). The psychology of worldviews. *Review of General Psychology, 8*(1), 3–58.

Kriesi, H. (2014). The populist challenge. *West European Politics, 37*(2), 361–378.

Kriesi, H., & Pappas, T. S. (2015). *European populism in the shadow of the great recession.* ECPR Press.

Kuhn, T. (1970). *The structure of scientific revolutions.* Chicago University Press.

Lakatos, I. (1978). *Methodology of scientific research communities* (J. Worrall & G. Currie, Eds.). Cambridge University Press.

Landau, M. J., Kay, A. C., & Whitson, J. A. (2015). Compensatory control and the appeal of a structured world. *Psychological Bulletin, 141*(3), 694–722. https://doi.org/10.1037/a0038703

Langs, R. (1974). *The technique of psychoanalytic psychotherapy.* Jason Aronson, Inc. (Original work published 1973)

Lepper, G. (2012). Taking a pragmatic approach to dialogical science. *International Journal of Dialogical Science, 6*(1), 149–159.

Lickliter, R., & Honeycutt, H. (2013). A developmental evolutionary framework for psychology. *Review of General Psychology, 17*, 184–189.

Ligorio, M. B. (2002). *Apprendimento e collaborazione in ambienti di realtà virtuale: Teoria, metodi, tecniche ed esperienze* [Learning and cooperation in virtual environmental: Theory, methods, techniques and experiences]. Garamond.

Lindblom, C. E. (1959). The science of "muddling through". *Public Administration, 19*, 79–88.

Lindblom, J. (2015). *Embodied social cognition.* Springer.

Linell, P. (2009). *Rethinking language, mind and world dialogically: Interactional and contextual theories of sense-making.* Information Age Publishing.

Lingiardi, V. (2002). *L'alleanza terapeutica: Teoria, clinica, ricerca* [The therapeutic alliance: Theory, clinic and research]. Raffaello Cortina.

Madeo, D., Salvatore, S., Mannarini, T., & Mocenni, C. (2021). Modeling pluralism and self-regulation explains the emergence of cooperation in networked societies. *Scientific Reports, 11*, 19226.

Mandler, G. (2011). From association to organization. *Current Directions in Psychological Science, 20*, 232–235.

Mannarini, T., Rochira, A., Ciavolino, E., Russo, F., & Salvatore, S. (2020). The demand for populism: A psycho-cultural based analysis of the desire for non mainstream political representation. *Psychology Hub, 37*(2), 31–39.

Mannarini, T., Rochira, A., Ciavolino, E., & Salvatore, S. (2019). Individual and community determinants of sense of community: The role of universalistic values. *Journal of Community Psychology*, 1–15.

Mannarini, T., Veltri, A. G., & Salvatore, S. (Eds.). (2020). *Media and social representations of otherness. Psycho-social-cultural implications.* Springer.

Manzotti, R. (2010). There are no images (to be seen) or the fallacy of the intermediate entity. *APA Newsletter on Philosophy and Computers, 9*, 59–66.

Marinaci, T., Venuleo, C., Ferrante, L., & Della Bona, S. (2021). What game we are playing: The psychosocial context of problem gambling, problem gaming and poor well-being among Italian high school students. *Heliyon, 7*(8), e07872.

Mariotti, S. (1995). Flessibilità: Lezioni e limiti della lean production [Flexibility: Lessions and limits of the lean production]. *Economia & Management, 2,* 30–43.

Markova, I. (2003). *Dialogicality and social representations: The dynamics of mind.* Cambridge University Press.

Marr, D. (1982). *Vision: A computational investigation into the human representation and processing of visual information.* Freeman.

Marsh, T., & Boag, S. (2014). Unifying psychology: Shared ontology and the continuum of practical assumptions. *Review of General Psychology, 18,* 49–59.

Matte Blanco, I. (1975). *The unconscious as infinite sets: An essays in bi-logic.* Gerald Duckworth and Co. Ltd.

Maturana, M. R., & Varela, J. F. (1980). *Autopoiesis and cognition: The realization of the living.* Reidel Publishing Co.

Mazzoni, G. (2015). *I destini generali* [General destines]. Laterza Editore.

McNamee, S., & Gergen, K. J. (Eds.). (1992). *Therapy as social construction.* Sage Publishing.

Mead, M. (1928). *Coming on age in Samoa.* William Morrow and Company.

Melchert, T. P. (2016). Leaving behind our preparadigmatic past: Professional psychology as a unified clinical science. *American Psychologist, 71*(6), 486–496.

Montesarchio, G., & Venuleo, C. (2010). *Gruppo esclamativo* [Exclamative group]. Franco Angeli.

Moscovici, S. (1976). *La psychanalyse son image et son public: Etude sur la répresentation sociale de la psychanalyse.* Presses Universitaires de France. (Original work published 1961) [English edition by Duveen, G. (2008). *Psychoanalysis: Its image and its public.* Polity Press].

Mossi, P., Ingusci, E., Tonti, M., & Salvatore, S. (2019). QUASUS: A tool for measuring the parents' school satisfaction. *Frontiers of Psychology, 10,* 13. https://doi.org/10.3389/fpsyg.2019.00013

Mudde, C. (2004). The populist zeitgeist. *Government and Opposition, 39*(4), 541–563. https://doi.org/10.1111/j.1477-7053.2004.00135.x

Muller, J. P. (1996). *Beyond the psychoanalytic dyad: Developmental semiotics in Freud, Peirce and Lacan.* Routledge.

Neisser, U. (1976). *Cognition and reality.* Freeman.

Newman, K. L. (2000). Organizational transformation during institutional upheaval. *Academy of Management Review, 25,* 602.

Norman, R. (1986). *Service management: Strategy and leadership in service businesses.* Wiley.

Nowell, B., & Boyd, N. M. (2014). Sense of community responsibility in community collaboratives: Advancing a theory of community resource and responsibility. *American Journal of Community Psychology, 54,* 229–242.

Orlinsky, D. E., Rønnestad, M. H., & Willutzki, U. (2004). Fifty years of psychotherapy process-outcome research: Continuity and change. In M. J. Lambert (Ed.), *Bergin and Garfield's handbook of psychotherapy and behavior change* (5th ed., pp. 309–390). Wiley.

Osgood, C. E., May, W. H., & Miron, M. S. (1975). *Cross-cultural universals of affective meaning.* Illinois University Press.

Osgood, C. E., Suci, G. J., & Tannenbaum, P. H. (1957). *The measurement of meaning.* Illinois University Press.

Paniccia, R. M., & Salvatore, S. (1998). Il colloquio: Dalla tecnica all'intervento [The interview: From the technique to the intervention]. In G. Montesarchio (a cura di), *Colloquio da manuale* (pp. 77–113). Giuffrè Editore.

Peirce, C. S. (1932a). Harvard lecture on pragmatism. In C. Hartshorne & P. Weiss (Eds.), *Collected papers of Charles Sanders Peirce* (Vol. II). Harvard University Press. (Original work published 1902)

Peirce, C. S. (1932b). On sign. In C. Hartshorne & P. Weiss (Eds.), *Collected papers of Charles Sanders Peirce* (Vol. II). Harvard University Press. (Original work published 1897)

Peirce, C. S. (1976). Application to the Carnegie institution. In C. Eisele (Ed.), *The new elements of mathematics by Charles S. Peirce*. Mouton Publishers. (Original work published 1902)

Perret-Clermont, A.-N., Pontecorvo, C., Resnick, L. B., Zittoun, T., & Burge, B. (Eds.). (2004). *Joining society: Social interaction and learning in adolescence and youth*. Cambridge University Press.

Pessa, E., & Penna, M. P. (2000). *Manuale di scienza cognitiva: Intelligenza artificiale e psicologia cognitiva* [Handbook of cognitive science: Artificial intelligence and cognitive psychology]. Editori Laterza.

Peterson, J. B., & Flanders, J. L. (2002). Complexity management theory: Motivation for ideological rigidity and social conflict. *Cortex: A Journal Devoted to the Study of the Nervous System and Behavior, 38*(3), 429–458. https://doi.org/10.1016/S0010-9452(08)70680-4

Peterson, N. A., Speer, P. W., & McMillan, D. W. (2008). Validation of a brief sense of community scale: Confirmation of the principal theory of sense of community. *Journal of Community Psychology, 1*, 61–73.

Piaget, J. (1936). *Origins of intelligence in the child*. Routledge & Kegan Paul.

Piketty, T. (2014). *Capital in the twenty-first century*. Harvard University Press. (Original work published by Editions du Seuil 2013)

Poggiani, F. (2012). What makes a reasoning sound? C. D. Peirce's normative foundation of logics. *Transactions of the Charles S. Peirce Society: A Quarterly Journal in American Philosophy, 48*(1), 31–50.

Pontecorvo, C. (1990). Social context, semiotic mediation, and forms of discourse in constructing knowledge at school. In H. Mandl, E. De Corte, S. N. Bennett, & H. F. Friedrich (a cura di), *Learning and instruction: European research in an international context* (pp. 1–26). Pergamon Press.

Proulx, T., & Inzlicht, M. (2012). The five "A"s of meaning maintenance: Finding meaning in the theories of sense-making. *Psychological Inquiry, 23*(4), 317–335.

Putnam, R. D. (2000). *Bowling alone: The collapse and revival of American community*. Simon & Schuster.

Ratner, C. (2008). Cultural psychology and qualitative methodology: Scientific and political considerations. *Culture & Psychology, 14*(3), 259–288.

Re.Cri.Re. Consortium. (2018). *TR-design of general criteria for policy making*. Deliverable 5.1 del Progetto Re.Cri.Re. www.recrire.eu

Rocco, D., Gennaro, A., Salvatore, S., Stoycheva, V., & Bucci, W. (2017). Clinical mutual attunement and the development of therapeutic process: A preliminary study. *Journal of Constructivist Psychology, 30*(4), 371–387. https://doi.org/10.1080/10720537.2016.1227950

Rochira, A., Guidi, M., Mannarini, T., & Salvatore, S. (2015). The representations of teachers' role identity: A study on the "professional common sense". *Rivista di Psicologia Clinica, 10*(1), 94–130. www.rivistadipsicologiaclinica.it

Rochira, A., Mannarini, T., Fini, V., & Salvatore, S. (2019). Symbolic universes, semiotic capital and health. A semiotic cultural psychological analysis of the vaccination hesitancy phenomenon in Italy. In S. Salvatore, V. Fini, T. Mannarini, J. Valsiner, & G. A. Veltri (Eds.), *Symbolic universes in time of (post)crisis: The future of European societies* (pp. 215–233). Springer.

Russo, F., Mannarini, T., & Salvatore, S. (2020). From the manifestations of culture to the underlying sensemaking process: The contribution of semiotic cultural psychology theory to the interpretation of socio-political scenario. *Journal for the Theory of Social Behaviour, 50*(3), 301–320.

Safran, J. D., & Muran, J. C. (2000). *Negotiating the therapeutic alliance: A relational treatment guide*. Guildford Press.

Salgado, J., & Clegg, J. W. (2011). Dialogism and the psyche: Bakhtin and contemporary psychology. *Culture & Psychology, 17*(4), 421–440.

Salvatore, S. (2001). *La scuola come cliente* [The school as client]. Franco Angeli.

Salvatore, S. (2006). Models of knowledge and psychological action. *Rivista di Psicologia Clinica, 1*(2–3). www.rivistapsicologiaclinica.it

Salvatore, S. (2012). Social life of the sign: Sensemaking in society. In J. Valsiner (Ed.), *The Oxford handbook of culture and psychology* (pp. 241–254). Oxford University Press.

Salvatore, S. (2013). The reciprocal inherency of self and context: Outline for a semiotic model of constitution of experience. *Interacções, 24*(9), 20–50. www.eses.pt/interaccoes

Salvatore, S. (2014). The mountain of cultural psychology and the mouse of empirical studies: Methodological considerations for birth control. *Culture & Psychology, 20*(4), 477–500.

Salvatore, S. (2016a). *L'intervento psicologico: Teoria e metodo della funzione psicologica* [The psychological intervention: Theory and method of the psychological function]. Edizioni Carlo Amore – Firera Publishing Group Bruner (Original work published 1990).

Salvatore, S. (2016b). The contingent nature of psychological intervention: From blind spot to basic resource of psychological science. In G. Sammut, J. Foster, S. Salvatore, & R. Andrisano-Ruggieri (Eds.), *Methods of psychological intervention: Yearbook of idiographic science series* (Vol. 7, pp. 13–54). Information Age Publishing.

Salvatore, S. (2016c). *Psychology in black and white: The project of a theory-driven science*. Information Age Publishing.

Salvatore, S. (2017). The formalization of cultural psychology: Reasons and functions. *Integrative Psychological and Behavioral Science, 51*(1), 1–13. https://doi.org/10.1007/s12124-016-9366-2

Salvatore, S. (2018). Cultural psychology as the science of sensemaking: A semiotic-cultural framework for psychology. In A. Rosa & J. Valsiner (Eds.), *The Cambridge handbook of sociocultural psychology* (2nd ed., pp. 35–48). Cambridge University Press.

Salvatore, S. (2019a). Lotteries, bets, Coca-Cola and Octopus Paul: The extraordinary of ordinary. In G. Marsico & L. Tateo (Eds.), *Ordinary things and their extraordinary meanings* (pp. 123–144). Information Age Publishing.

Salvatore, S. (2019b). Beyond the meaning given: The meaning as explanandum. *Integrative Psychological and Behavioural Science, 53*, 632–643.

Salvatore, S. (2021a). Ideas and challenges for cultural psychology. In B. Wagoner, B. A. Christensen, & C. Demuth (Eds.), *Culture as process* (pp. 355–362). Springer.

Salvatore, S. (2021b). Una critica alla definizione in positivo della salute [A critique to the positive definition of health]. *Psicologia della Salute, 2*, 35–39.

Salvatore, S., Ando', A., Ruggieri, R. A., Bucci, F., Cordella, B., Freda, M. F., Lombardo, C., Lo Coco, G., Novara, C., Petito, A., Schimmenti, A., Vegni, E., Venuleo, C., Zagaria, A., & Zennaro, A. (2022). Compartmentalization and unity of professional psychology: A road map for the future of the discipline. *Rivista di Psicologia Clinica, 1*(1–29). https://doi.org/10.3280/rpc1-2022oa14450

Salvatore, S., Avdi, E., Battaglia, F., Bernal-Marcos, M., Buhagiar, L. J., Ciavolino, E., Fini, V., Kadianaki, I., Kullasepp, K., Mannarini, T., Matsopoulos, A., Mossi, P. G., Rochira, A., Sammut, G., Santarpia, A., & Veltri, G. A. (2019a). Distribution and characteristics of symbolic universes over the European societies. In S. Salvatore, V. Fini, T. Mannarini, J. Valsiner, & G. A. Veltri (Eds.), *Symbolic universes in time of (post)crisis: The future of European societies* (pp. 135–170). Springer.

Salvatore, S., Avdi, E., Battaglia, F., Bernal-Marcos, M., Buhagiar, L. J., Ciavolino, E., Fini, V., Kadianaki, I., Kullasepp, K., Mannarini, T., Matsopoulos, A., Mossi, P. G., Rochira, A., Sammut, G., Santarpia, A., Veltri, G. A., & Valmorbida, A. (2019b). The cultural milieu and the symbolic universes of European societies. In S. Salvatore, V. Fini, T. Mannarini, J. Valsiner, & G. A. Veltri (Eds.), *Symbolic universes in time of (post)crisis: The future of European societies* (pp. 53–133). Springer.

Salvatore, S., De Luca Picione, R., Cozzolino, M., Bochicchio, V., & Palmieri, A. (2022). The role of affective sensemaking in the constitution of experience: The affective pertinentization model (APER). *Integrative Psychological and Behavioral Science, 56*(1), 114–132.

Salvatore, S., Fini, V., Mannarini, T., Veltri, G. A., Avdi, E., Battaglia, F., Castro-Tejerina, J., Ciavolino, E., Cremaschi, M., Kadianaki, I., Kharlamov, A. N., Krasteva, A., Kullasepp, K., Matsopoulos, A., Meschiari, C., Mossi, P., Psinas, P., Redd, R., Rochira, A., . . . Valmorbida, A. (2018). Symbolic universes between present and future of Europe: First results of the map of European societies' cultural milieu. *PLOS One, 13*(1), e0189885.

Salvatore, S., Forges Davanzati, G., Potì, S., & Ruggeri, R. (2009). Mainstream economics and sense-making. *Integrative Psychological and Behavioral Science, 43*(2), 158–177.

Salvatore, S., & Freda, M. F. (2011). Affect unconscious and sensemaking: A psychodynamic semiotic and dialogic model. *New Ideas in Psychology, 29*, 119–135.

Salvatore, S., Freda, M. F., Ligorio, B., Iannaccone, A., Rubino, F., Scotto di Carlo, M., Bastianoni, P., & Gentile, M. (2003). Socioconstructivism and theory of the unconscious: A gaze over a research horizon. *European Journal of School Psychology, 1*(1), 9–36.

Salvatore, S., Gelo, O., Gennaro, A., & Manzo, S. (2010). Looking at the psychotherapy process as an intersubjective dynamic of meaning-making: A case study with discourse flow analysis. *Journal of Constructivist Psychology, 23*(3), 195–230.

Salvatore, S., & Gennaro, A. (2015). Outlines of a general semiotic and dynamic theory of the psychotherapy process: The clinical exchange as communicational field: Theoretical considerations and methodological implications. In O. Gelo, A. Pritz, & B. Rieken (Eds.), *Psychotherapy research* (pp. 195–212). Springer.

Salvatore, S., Ligorio, M. B., & De Franchis, C. (2005). Does psychoanalytic theory have anything to say on learning? *European Journal of School Psychology, 3*(1), 101–126.

Salvatore, S., Mannarini, T., Avdi, E., Battaglia, F., Cremaschi, M., Forges Davanzati, G., Fini, V., Kadianaki, I., Krasteva, A., Matsopoulos, A., Mølholm, M., Redd, R.,

Rochira, A., Russo, F., Santarpia, A., Sammut, G., Valmorbida, A., & Veltri, G. A. (2019). Globalization, demand of sense and enemization of the other: A psycho-cultural analysis of European societies' socio-political crisis. *Culture & Psychology, 25*(3), 345–374.

Salvatore, S., Mannarini, T., Gennaro, A., Celia, G., De Dominicis, S., De Luca Picione, R., Iuso, S., Kerusauskaite, S., Kleinbub, J. R., Pergola, F., Reho, M., Rochira, R., & Rocchi, G. (2023). The affective regulation of uncertainty: The semiotic dimensionality model (SDM). *Social Sciences, 12*, 217. https://doi.org/10.3390/socsci12040217

Salvatore, S., Palmieri, A., Cordella, B., & Iuso, S. (2021). The decay of signs' semi-otic value: A cultural psychology interpretation of the contemporary social scenario. *Culture & Psychology, 27*(4), 539–561.

Salvatore, S., Sanchez-Cardenas, M., De Luca Picione, R., & Pergola, F. (submitted). *Psychoanalysis in a semiotic key: Implications for theory, theory of technique, and clinical practice.*

Salvatore, S., & Scotto di Carlo, M. (2005). *L'intervento psicologico per la scuola: Modelli, metodi, strumenti* [The psychological intervention for the school. Models, methods, tools]. Edizioni Carlo Amore – Firera Publishing Group.

Salvatore, S., Tebaldi, C., & Poti, S. (2009). The discursive dynamic of sensemaking. In S. Salvatore, J. Valsiner, S. Strout, & J. Clegg (Eds.), *Yearbook of idiographic science* (Vol. 1, pp. 39–72). Firera Publishing Group. (Original work published 2006, *International Journal of Idiographic Science*, Article 3 [online journal]).

Salvatore, S., Tonti, M., & Gennaro, A. (2017). How to model sensemaking: A contribution for the development of a methodological framework for the analysis of meaning. In M. Han & C. Cunha (Eds.), *The subjectified and subjectifying mind* (pp. 245–268). Information Age Publishing.

Salvatore, S., & Tschacher, W. (2012). Time dependency of psychotherapeutic exchanges: The contribution of the theory of dynamic systems in analyzing process. *Frontiers in Psychology, 3*, 253.

Salvatore, S., & Valsiner, J. (2009). Idiographic science on its way: Towards making sense of psychology. In S. Salvatore, J. Valsiner, S. Strout, & J. Clegg (Eds.), *Yearbook of idiographic science* (Vol. 1, pp. 9–19). Firera Publishing Group.

Salvatore, S., & Valsiner, J. (2010). Between the general and the unique: Overcoming the nomothetic versus idiographic opposition. *Theory and Psychology, 20*(6), 817–833.

Salvatore, S., & Valsiner, J. (2014). Outline of a general psychological theory of the psychological intervention. *Theory and Psychology, 24*, 217–232.

Salvatore, S., Valsiner, J., & Veltri, G. A. (2019). The theoretical and methodological framework. Semiotic cultural psychology, symbolic universes and lines of semiotic forces. In S. Salvatore, V. Fini, T. Mannarini, J. Valsiner, & G. A. Veltri (Eds.), *Symbolic universes in time of (post)crisis: The future of European societies* (pp. 25–49). Springer.

Salvatore, S., & Venuleo, C. (2013). Field dependency and contingency in the modeling of sensemaking. *Papers on Social Representation, 22*(2), 21.1–21.41 [online journal]

Salvatore, S., & Venuleo, C. (2017). Liminal transition in semiotic key: The mutual in-feeding between present and past. *Theory & Psychology, 27*, 215–230.

Salvatore, S., & Zittoun, T. (2011). Outlines of a psychoanalytically informed cultural psychology. In S. Salvatore & T. Zittoun (Eds.), *Cultural psychology and psychoanalysis in dialogue: Issues for constructive theoretical and methodological synergies* (pp. 3–46). Information Age Publication.

Sammut, G., Andreouli, E., Gaskell, G., & Valsiner, J. (Eds.). (2016). *The Cambridge handbook of social representations*. Cambridge University Press.

Sandler, J., & Dreher, A. U. (1996). *What do psychoanalysts want? The problem of aims in the psychoanalytic therapy*. Routledge.

Sapir, E. (1921). *Language: An introduction to the study of speech*. Harcourt, Brace & World Inc.

Sbisà, M. (2002). Presupposizioni e contesti [Presuppositions and contexts]. In C. Penco (a cura di), *La svolta contestuale* (pp. 221–239). McGraw Hill.

Scharfbilling, M., Smillie, L., Mair, D., Sienkiewicz, M., Keimer, J., Pinho Dos Santos, R., Vinagreiro Alves, H., Vecchione, E., & Scheunermann, L. (2021). *Values and identities – a policymakers' guide* (EUR 30800 EN). Publication Office of the European Union. ISBN 978-92-76-40966-2.

Schein, E. H. (1999). *The corporate culture survival guide*. John Wiley & Sons.

Schore, A. N. (2001). Minds in the making: Attachment, the self-organizing brain, and developmentally-oriented psychoanalytic psychotherapy. *British Journal of Psychotherapy*, *17*(3), 299–328.

Schwartz, S. H., Caprara, G. V., & Vecchione, M. (2010). Basic personal values, core political values, and voting: A longitudinal analysis. *Political Psychology*, *31*, 421–452. https://doi.org/10.1111/j.1467-9221.2010.00764.x

Schwartz, S. J. (2016). Basic individual values: Sources and consequences. In T. Brosch & D. Sander (Eds.), *Handbook of value: Perspectives from economics, neuroscience, philosophy, psychology and sociology* (pp. 63–62). Oxford University Press.

Seganti, A. (1998). *La memoria sensoriale delle relazioni: Ipotesi verificabili di psicoterapia psicoanalitica* [The sensorial memory of relationships: Verifiable hypotheses of psychoanaltytic psychoterapy]. Boringhieri.

Shweder, R. A. (1991). *Thinking through cultures: Expeditions in cultural psychology*. Harvard University Press.

Smedslund, J. (1988). *Psycho-logic*. Springer-Verlag.

Smorti, A., & Fioretti, C. (2019). Beyond the anomaly: Where Piaget and Bruner meet. *Integrative Psychological and Behavioral Science*, *53*, 694–706.

Sorrentino, P. (regista). (2021). *È stata la mano di Dio* [The hand of God]. The Apartment, Fremantle.

Stam, H. J. (2004). Unifying psychology: Epistemological act or disciplinary maneuver? *Journal of Clinical Psychology*, *60*, 1259–1262.

Steg, L., & Rothengatter, T. (2017). Introduction to applied psychology. In L. Steg, K. Keizer, A. P. Buunk, & T. Rothengatter (Eds.), *Applied social psychology: Understanding and managing social problems* (2nd ed., pp. 1–26). Cambridge University Press.

Stenner, P. (2017). *Liminality and experience: A transdisciplinary approach to the psychosocial*. Palgrave.

Stern, B. D. (2013a). Field theory in psychoanalysis, part I: Harry Stack Sullivan and Madeleine and Willy Baranger. *Psychoanalytic Dialogues*, *23*(5), 487–501.

Stern, B. D. (2013b). Field theory in psychoanalysis, part 2: Bionian field theory and contemporary interpersonal/relational psychoanalysis. *Psychoanalytic Dialogues*, *23*(6), 630–645.

Stern, D. N. (1985). *The interpersonal world of the infant*. Basic Books.

Stern, D. N. (2004). *The present moment in psychotherapy and everyday life*. W. W. Norton & Co.

Stolorow, R. D., Orange, D. M., & Atwood, G. E. (2001). World horizons: A post-cartesian alternative to the Freudian unconscious. *Contemporary Psychoanalysis*, *37*(1), 43–61.

Swendsen, G. T., & Swendsen, G. L. H. (Eds.). (2009). *Handbook of social capital: The Troika of sociology, political science and economics*. Edward Elgar Publishing.

Tajfel, H., & Turner, J. (1986). The social identity theory of intergroup relations. In S. Worchel & W. Austin (Eds.), *Psychology of intergroup relations* (2nd ed., pp. 7–17). Nelson-Hall.

Thompson, R. C., & Hunt, J. G. (1996). Inside the black box of alpha, beta, and gamma change: Using a cognitive-processing model to assess attitude structure. *Academy of Management Review*, *21*, 655–690.

Thornton, T. (2008). Should comprehensive diagnosis include idiographic under-standing? *Medical Health Care and Philosophy*, *11*, 293–302.

Tonti, M., & Salvatore, S. (2015). The homogenization of classification functions measurement (HOCFUN): A method for measuring the salience of emotional arousal in thinking. *American Journal of Psychology*, *128*(4), 469–483.

Toomela, A. (2007). Culture of science: Strange history of the methodological think-ing in psychology. *Integrative Psychological and Behavioral Science*, *41*(1), 6–20.

Toomela, A., & Valsiner, J. (2010). *Methodological thinking in psychology: 60 years gone astray?* Information Age Publishing.

Trandis, H. C., Bontempo, R., Villareal, M. J., Asai, M., & Lucca, N. (1988). Indi-vidualism and collectivism: Cross-cultural perspectives on self-ingroup relationships. *Journal of Personality and Social Psychology*, *54*(2), 323–338.

Trevarthen, C. (1998). The concept and foundations of infant intersubjectivity. *Inter-subjective Communication and Emotion in Early Ontogeny*, *15*, 46.

Trevarthen, C., & Aitken, K. J. (2001). Infant intersubjectivity: Research, theory, and clinical applications. *The Journal of Child Psychology and Psychiatry and Allied Dis-ciplines*, *42*(1), 3–48.

Tronick, E. (2007). *The neurobehavioral and social-emotional development of infants and children*. WW Norton & Company.

Tronick, E., & Beeghly, M. (2011). Infants' meaning-making and the development of mental health problems. *American Psychologist*, *66*(2), 107.

Valsiner, J. (2007). *Culture in minds and societies: Foundations of cultural psychology*. Sage Publishing.

Valsiner, J. (2009). Integrating psychology within the globalizing world: A requiem to the post-modernist experiment with Wissenschaft. *Integrative Psychological and Behavioral Science*, *43*(1), 1–21.

Valsiner, J. (2014). *An invitation to cultural psychology*. Sage Publishing.

Valsiner, J. (2020). *Sensuality in human living: The cultural psychology of affect*. Springer.

Valsiner, J., & Salvatore, S. (2012). How idiographic science could create its termi-nology? In S. Salvatore, J. Valsiner, & A. Gennaro (Eds.), *Making sense of infinite uniqueness: The emerging system of idiographic science yearbook of idiographic science* (Vol., 4, pp. 3–20). Information Age Publishing.

Valsiner, J., & Van der Veer, R. (2000). *The social mind: Construction of the idea*. Cam-bridge University Press.

van Dijk, T. A. (1998). *Ideology: A multidisciplinary approach*. Sage Publishing.

Veltri, G., Redd, R., Mannarini, T., & Salvatore, S. (2019). The identity of Brexit: A cultural psychology analysis. *Journal of Applied and Community Psychology*, *29*(1), 18–31.

Venezia, A., Mossi, P., Venuleo, C., Savarese, G., & Salvatore, S. (2019). Representations of physician's role and their impact on compliance. *Psicologia della Salute, 2,* 100–121.

Venuleo, C., Mossi, P. G., & Calogiuri, S. (2018). Combining cultural and individual dimensions in the analysis of hazardous behaviours: An explorative study on the interplay between cultural models, impulsivity and depression in hazardous drinking and gambling. *Journal of Gambling Issues, 40,* 69–115.

Venuleo, C., Mossi, P. G., & Salvatore, S. (2016). Educational subcultures and dropping out in higher education: A longitudinal case study. *Studies in Higher Education, 41*(2), 321–342. https://doi.org/10.1080/03075079.2014.927847

Venuleo, C., Salvatore, G., Andrisano Ruggieri, R., Marinaci, T., Cozzolino, M., & Salvatore, S. (2020). Steps towards a unified theory of psychopathology: The phase space of meaning model. *Clinical Neuropsychiatry, 17*(4), 236–252.

Venuleo, C., Salvatore, S., Mossi, P. G., Grassi, R., & Ruggieri, R. (2007). The teaching relationship in the changing world. Outlines for a theory of the reframing setting. *European Journal of School Psychology, 5*(2), 151–180.

Verheggen, T., & Baerveldt, C. B. (2007). "We don't share!" Exploring the theoretical ground for social and cultural psychology: The social representation approach versus an enactivism framework. *Culture & Psychology, 13*(1), 5–27.

Vygotsky, L. S. (1986). *Thought and language* (A. Kozulin, Rev. Ed.). MIT Press. (Original work published 1934)

Wagemans, J. (2018). Perceptual organization. In J. T. Wixed (Ed.), *Stevens' handbook of experimental psychology and cognitive neuroscience: Vol. 2. Sensation, perception, & attention* (pp. 803–872). Wiley & Sons.

Weick, K. (1995). *Sensemaking in organization.* Sage Publishing.

Westen, D., Morrison, K., & Thompson-Brenner, H. (2004). The empirical status of empirically supported psychotherapies: Assumptions, findings, and reporting in controlled clinical trials. *Psychological Bulletin, 130,* 631–663.

Windelband, W. (1998). History and natural science. *Theory & Psychology, 8*(1), 5–22. (Original speech 1894, German published version 1904)

Wittgenstein, L. (1958). *Philosophical investigations.* Basil Blackwell. (Original work published 1953)

World Bank. (2015). *World development report 2015: Mind, society, and behavior.* World Bank.

Zagaria, A., Andò, A., & Zennaro, A. (2020). Psychology: A giant with feet of clay. *Integrative Psychological and Behavioral Science, 54,* 521–562.

Zerubavel, E. (1999). *Social mindscapes: An invitation to cognitive sociology.* Harvard University Press.

Zimmerman, M. J. (2015). Value and normativity. In I. Hirose & J. Olson (Eds.), *The Oxford handbook of value theory* (pp. 13–28). Oxford University Press.

Zittoun, T. (2006). *Transitions.* Information Age Publishers.

Zucchermaglio, C. (2002). *Psicologia culturale dei gruppi* [Cultural group psycology]. Carocci.

INDEX